Anti-inflammatory Cookbook for Beginners

Quick and Easy Recipes to Detoxify and Rapidly Reduce Body Inflammation, Rebalance Hormones, and Strengthen the Immune System. Includes 31-Day Meal Plan.

By

ASTRID HINES

Table of Content

Introduction

Inflammation can shield the body from harm and improve the body's resistance to disease. Usually, it is a crucial stage in the healing process.

But in some people, an underlying medical condition prevents the immune system from functioning correctly. This malfunction may lead to low-grade inflammation that is persistent or recurrent.

A few of the disorders that result in chronic inflammation are asthma, rheumatoid arthritis, and psoriasis. There is evidence that altering one's diet can aid with symptom management.

Vegetables, fruits, meals high in fatty acids (omega-3), lean protein, whole grains, healthy fats, and spices are encouraged in anti-inflammatory diets. It discourages or limits the consumption of processed foods, alcohol, and red meat.

Instead of being a specific diet, an anti-inflammatory diet is more of a style of eating. Diets that reduce inflammation include DASH diet and Mediterranean diet, for example.

The majority of anti-inflammatory diet consists of fresh vegetables and fruits. Plant-based foods are rich in antioxidants. However, some substances can actually lead to the creation of free radicals. Examples include foods that are continuously fried in hot oil.

Food contains dietary antioxidant compounds that help the body remove free radicals. Free radicals are byproducts of various physiological processes, including metabolism, which occur naturally in the body. However, stress and smoking are two examples of external stressors that may increase the body's levels of free radicals.

Free radicals are capable of causing cell harm. This damage increases the likelihood of inflammation and may support many illnesses.

Dietary antioxidants help remove these toxic compounds in addition to the antioxidants the body naturally produces.

In anti-inflammatory diet, foods that reduce the production of free radicals are chosen above those that are high in antioxidants.

Chapter 1: Anti-inflammatory diet

The body can be protected from harm by inflammation, which also aids in the body's ability to fight disease. It is typically an essential step in the healing process.

The immune system, however, does not function normally in some persons due to a medical problem. An ongoing or repeated low level of inflammation may result from this dysfunction.

Asthma, rheumatoid arthritis, and psoriasis are just a few of the conditions that cause chronic inflammation. There is proof that changing one's diet can help manage symptoms.

Anti-inflammatory diet favors vegetables, fruits, omega-3-rich meals, lean protein, whole grains, healthy fats, and the spices. It restricts or discourages the consumption of alcohol, processed foods, and red meat.

An anti-inflammatory diet is more of a way of eating than a precise plan. Anti-inflammatory diets include DASH diet and Mediterranean diet, for instance.

1.1: What is anti-inflammatory diet?

Certain food items have the potential to either cause or exacerbate inflammation. Sugary or processed foods may cause this, although whole, fresh foods are much less likely to do so.

Fresh vegetables and fruits make up the bulk of anti-inflammatory diet. Antioxidants are abundant in plant-based meals. But some foods can actually cause the production of free radicals. Examples include dishes that are fried in continuously hot frying oil.

Dietary antioxidant substances are found in the food that assists body in the removal of free radicals. Free radicals are byproducts that are produced naturally by several body functions, including the metabolism. However, smoking and stress are examples of outside stressors that might raise the body's free radical levels.

Cell damage can be caused by free radicals. This harm raises the possibility of inflammation and can support a number of disorders.

In addition to the antioxidants produced naturally by the body, dietary antioxidants also aid in the removal of these harmful chemicals.

Foods high in the antioxidants are preferred over those that boost the generation of free radicals in an anti-inflammatory diet.

Fatty acids (Omega-3), which are found in the oily fish, may aid in lowering the body's levels of inflammatory proteins. Fiber can have similar results as well,

Benefits of anti-inflammatory diet

Oxidative stress, which is cell damage brought on by free radicals, can be defended against by antioxidants.

The following actions and procedures can result in oxidative stress:

- Excessive exercise
- Mitochondrial activity
- Tissue trauma, caused due to any injury and inflammation
- Smoking
- Ischemia and reperfusion damage
- Consumption of the certain food items, especially the processed and refined foods, artificial, trans fats
- ozone
- Sweeteners, with certain additives and dyes
- Radiation
- Environmental pollution
- Exposure to the chemicals, for example such as drugs and pesticides, including the chemotherapy
- industrial solvents

Cell damage may occur as a result of such exposures and activities.

- An excessive release of free iron or copper ions may result from this.
- A phagocyte activation, a type of white blood cell involved in infection defense.
- A rise in the number of free radical-producing enzymes.
- A break in the electron transport network.

Oxidative stress can be brought on by any of these.

Cancer, atherosclerosis, and eyesight loss have all been related to the harm done by oxidative stress. Free radicals are believed to alter cells, resulting in these and possibly other illnesses.

Antioxidant consumption is thought to lower these risks.

Who could it benefit?

Many illnesses that are made worse by chronic inflammation may benefit from anti-inflammatory diet like supplemental therapy.

Inflammation occurs in the following diseases:

Psoriasis

Rheumatoid arthritis

Asthma

Eosinophilic esophagitis

Colitis

Cohn's disease

The disease of inflammatory bowel

Hashimoto's thyroiditis

Lupus

Metabolic syndrome

Cardiovascular disease, obesity, diabetes type 2, and high rate blood pressure are only a few of the disorders referred to as the metabolic syndrome because they frequently co-occur.

Each of these, according to scientists, is impacted by inflammation. Therefore, a person with the metabolic syndrome may benefit from eating anti-inflammatory foods to improve their health.

Antioxidant-rich diets also may help lower the chance of developing some malignancies.

Using antioxidants can help eliminate free radicals.

1.2: Kinds of the anti-inflammatory diet

Anti-inflammatory tenets are already present in many famous diets.

For instance, DASH diet and Mediterranean diet both consist of whole grains, fish, fresh vegetables and fruits and heart-healthy fats.

Mediterranean diet, with its emphasis on the plant-based products and beneficial oils, may be able to reduce the impact of the inflammation on the cardiovascular system, according to studies. Inflammation appears to play a role in cardiovascular disease.

1.3: Foods to consume

A diet for reducing inflammation should include a wide range of foods that:

- Offer a variety of antioxidants
- Very healthy and rich in the nutrients
- Contain healthy fats

Among the foods which might reduce inflammation are:

Some oily fish, for example, such as salmon and tuna

Fruits, for example, such as blackberries, blueberries, cherries, and strawberries

Vegetables, such as including broccoli, spinach and kale

Seeds and nuts

Beans

Fiber

Olive oil and olives

Moderately cooked or raw vegetables

Spices, for example, such as turmeric and ginger

Legumes, like lentils

Tea

Prebiotics and probiotics

Some herbs

It's important to keep in mind that no one food can significantly improve health. A variety of nutritious ingredients should be present in the diet.

Ingredients should be basic and fresh. Foods' nutritional value can be altered during processing.

Premade food labels should be read by consumers. For instance, while cocoa could be an excellent option, items that incorporate cocoa frequently also have sugar and fat.

An array of antioxidants, as well as other nutrients, can be found on a colourful plate. Make sure to mix up the hues of your vegetables and fruits.

13 Best Foods for Reducing inflammation

Inflammation has both beneficial and harmful effects.

On the one side, it assists the body in protecting itself against infection and damage.

However, persistent inflammation can result in disease.

This risk may increase as a result of stress, inactivity, and inflammatory meals.

But research indicates that some meals may help reduce chronic inflammation.

These 13 foods help to reduce inflammation.

1. **Berries:**

Berries are a type of tiny fruit rich in vitamins, fibre, and minerals.

There are dozens of variations. Strawberries, raspberries, blueberries, and blackberries are a few of the most popular.

Anthocyanins, an antioxidant found in berries, are present. The anti-inflammatory properties of these substances may lower your chance of developing a disease.

In one experiment with 25 adults, those who regularly ingested blueberry powder produced noticeably more naturally occurring killer cells (NK cells) than those who did not. These results agreed with those of an earlier investigation.

NK cells are produced by your body naturally, and they aid in maintaining a healthy immune system.

Another study found that eating strawberries reduced specific inflammatory markers linked to the heart disease in overweight persons compared to those who did not.

2. **Fatty fish**

The long-chain fatty acids (omega-3) (EPA), eicosapentaenoic acid and the docosahexaenoic acid, which are found in the fatty fish, are excellent sources of protein (DHA).

The following fatty fish are among the finest sources of omega-3 fatty acids, even though all varieties of fish contain some of them:

Salmon

Anchovies

Sardines

Mackerel

Herring

By reducing inflammation, EPA and DHA protect against metabolic syndrome, heart disease, diabetes, and renal disease.

Protectins and resolvins, which have anti-inflammatory properties, are produced by your body's metabolism of these fatty acids.

C-reactive protein levels were shown to decrease in those who consumed salmon or EPA and DHA supplementation, according to studies (CRP).

But in one trial, those with an irregular heartbeat who took EPA and DHA daily had no difference in their inflammatory markers compared to those who received a placebo.

3. Broccoli

Broccoli is a very wholesome vegetable.

Along with cauliflower, kale, and the brussels sprouts, it belongs to the cruciferous vegetable family.

Consuming a lot of cruciferous veggies is linked to a lower risk of cancer and heart disease, according to research.

The antioxidants they contain may have anti-inflammatory impact, which could explain this.

Sulforaphane, one of the antioxidant is found in abundance in the broccoli, which reduces the inflammation from lowering up body's levels of the (NF-B) nuclear factor kappa B and cytokines, chemicals that cause inflammation.

4. Avocados

Avocados are a powerhouse of fibre, monounsaturated fatty acids, potassium, and magnesium.

Additionally, they have tocopherols and carotenoids, which have been associated with a lower risk of the cancer.

In addition, a component in avocados may lessen inflammation in the skin cells that are still developing.

Interleukin 1 beta (IL-1 beta) and CRP, two inflammatory indicators, decreased in 51 overweight persons who consumed avocado for twelve weeks for one rising study.

5. **Green tea**

You've probably heard that one of the healthiest drinks you can consume is green tea.
Its consumption has been linked to a lower risk of the heart disease, Alzheimer's disease, cancer, obesity, and some other illnesses, according to research.
Several of its health advantages stem from its anti-inflammatory and antioxidant capabilities, particularly those of a compound called (EGCG) epigallocatechin-3-gallate.
By lowering the generation of pro-inflammatory cytokines and preventing damage to the fatty acids in your cells, EGCG prevents inflammation.

6. **Peppers**

The antioxidants and vitamin C found in chilli peppers, and bell peppers have potent anti-inflammatory properties.
The antioxidant quercetin, which is present in bell peppers and may help to lessen inflammation linked to chronic conditions like diabetes.
Because of the presence of ferulic acid and sinapic acid in the chilli peppers, these compounds may support

7. **Mushrooms**

Although there are thousands of different kinds of mushrooms, only a small number are edible and are raised economically.
These include portobello mushrooms, shiitake mushrooms, and truffles.
Selenium, copper, and all of the B vitamins are abundant in mushrooms, which also provide very few calories.
They also have additional antioxidants, such as phenols, that protect against inflammation.
Lion's mane, a unique variety of mushrooms, may be able to lessen obesity-related low-grade inflammation.
But according to one study, boiling mushrooms drastically reduced the anti-inflammatory chemicals in them. Therefore, it could be best to eat them raw or very briefly cooked.

8. Grapes

The anti-inflammatory compound anthocyanins are found in grapes.

They may also lower the risk of developing a number of illnesses, including diabetes, Alzheimer's, obesity, and eye conditions, as well as the heart disease and some other conditions.

Another antioxidant component with numerous health advantages, resveratrol, is likewise best found in grapes.

Resveratrol has been shown in studies to be able to guard the heart against inflammation. 60 heart failure patients participated in a trial where those who took two 50-mg resveratrol capsules daily for three months saw a reduction in inflammatory gene markers, including interleukin 6 (IL-6).

Adults who regularly ate grape extract had higher levels of the hormone adiponectin, according to an older study from 2012. Cancer risk and weight gain are both correlated with low levels of this hormone.

9. Turmeric

A common spice used in the curries as well as other Indian cuisines, turmeric has a warm, earthy flavour.

Due to the presence of curcumin, a potent anti-inflammatory substance, has drawn a lot of interest.

Turmeric has been found in studies to lessen inflammation brought on by diabetes, arthritis, and other disorders.

People who had metabolic syndrome in one trial took piperine from black pepper along with 1 g of the curcumin daily. The CRP inflammatory marker significantly dropped in these people.

It could be challenging to obtain enough curcumin from the turmeric on its own to feel a meaningful effect. It can be considerably more effective to take pills with isolated curcumin.

Piperine, which can increase curcumin absorption by 2000%, is frequently used in curcumin supplements.

To fully comprehend how turmeric dosage impacts inflammatory indicators, more research is required.

10. olive oil (Extra virgin)

Among the healthiest types of fat to consume is olive oil (extra virgin).
It is a mainstay of a Mediterranean diet and high in monounsaturated fats that have many positive health effects.
Olive oil (extra virgin) is associated with a lower risk of heart disease, brain cancer, and other major health issues, according to studies.
CRP and the number of other inflammatory markers were decreased in one trial on the Mediterranean diet in those who drank 1.7 ounces (50 mL) of olive oil daily for twelve months.
Oleocanthal, another antioxidant included in olive oil, has been shown to have similar anti-inflammatory effects to ibuprofen.
Always remember that olive oil (extra virgin) has superior anti-inflammatory properties over processed olive oil.

11. Dark chocolate and cocoa

Rich, gratifying, and tasty dark chocolates are available.
Additionally, it is abundant in antioxidants, which aid to lessen inflammation. These could lessen your risk of getting sick and promote healthier ageing.
The anti-inflammatory properties of chocolate are due to flavanols, which also support the health of the endothelial cells that are lining your arteries.
One tiny study found that after two weeks of consuming 350 mg of cocoa flavanols twice a day, vascular function had improved.
More thorough research on chocolate and its constituent parts is nonetheless required.
To gain these anti-inflammatory advantages in the meanwhile, it can't harm to select dark chocolate, which has at least 70 per cent cocoa—a higher percentage is much better.

12. Tomatoes

The tomatoes are the powerhouse of nutrients.
Vitamin C, potassium, and lycopene, an antioxidant with potent anti-inflammatory qualities, are all abundant in tomatoes.
Lycopene may be especially helpful for lowering pro-inflammatory substances linked to certain cancer types.

You should be aware that cooking tomatoes in olive oil can increase your absorption of the lycopene they contain.
This is so because lycopene is carotenoid, a type of nutrient that is more easily absorbed when combined with a supply of fat.

13. Cherries

Cherries are sweet and full of antioxidants like catechins and anthocyanins, which reduce inflammation.
Sweet cherries also have health benefits, albeit tart cherries have been the subject of more research than other types.
According to one study including 37 senior citizens, those who drank 16 ounces (480 mL) of sour cherry juice every day for 12 weeks saw considerably reduced levels of the inflammatory marker CRP.
However, a different study discovered that after taking tart cherry juice every day for thirty days, healthy young adults showed no effect on inflammation.

1.4: Foods to Avoid

People who are following an anti-inflammatory diet should avoid or limit their intake of:
Foods that have added salt and sugar or salt
Processed foods
Processed carbs that are found the white bread, puff pastry, white pasta and many other baking
Oils that are unhealthy
A processed snack such as crackers and chips
Heavy amount of alcohol
Ready-to-eat desserts like candy, marshmallows, cookies and ice cream
In addition, many people might find out it helpful to limit up their consumption of following:
Gluten: When they do consume gluten, some people develop an inflammatory response. It's not ideal for everyone to follow a gluten-free diet because it might be limiting.

However, if someone believes gluten is bringing on their symptoms, they might want to think about cutting it out for a period to see if their condition gets better.

Nightshades: Some persons with inflammatory disorders appear to experience flare-ups when consuming plants from nightshade families, such as eggplants, tomatoes, peppers, and the potatoes. A person can try eliminating nightshades from their diet for two to three weeks to see if their symptoms get better, though there isn't much data to support this impact.

Carbohydrates: There has been some evidence to suggest that some individuals may experience inflammatory promotion from a high-carb diet, even when the carbs are healthy. However, some meals high in carbohydrates, such as healthy grains and sweet potatoes, are great sources of antioxidants and other minerals.

Can a vegetarian diet reduce inflammation?

If someone wants to lessen inflammation, they can consider being vegetarian. Data from 40 research were evaluated by the authors of a 2019 review. They came to the conclusion that those who consume a vegetarian diet are probably to have lower levels of a number of inflammatory indicators.

In a 2017 survey, the information of 268 participants who either adhered to a rigid vegetarian diet, vegetarian diet (a Lacto-ovo), or a nonvegetarian diet was examined. According to the research, eating animal products can make you more likely to develop insulin resistance and systemic inflammation.

Lower levels of inflammation may be a major advantage of a vegan diet, according to earlier studies from 2014.

Tips for Anti-inflammatory diet

Changing one's eating habits might be difficult. However, the following advice may be helpful:

- When you go shopping once a week, stock up on a variety of veggies, fruits, and healthy snacks.
- Gradually substitute wholesome, homemade lunches for fast food dinners.
- Use still or sparkling mineral water in place of soda and other sugary drinks.

Talking to a doctor about dietary supplements like cod liver oil or a multivitamin is another suggestion.

- Including thirty min of brisk activity in the daily schedule.

• Adopting proper sleep hygiene, as little sleep can make inflammation worse.

1.5: A 21 days Meal plan

Day: 1

Breakfast: Spinach & Egg Scramble with Raspberries

Drinks: Chocolate Nutter Butter Smoothie

Lunch: Caprese Snack Skewers

Snacks: Chocolate-Peanut Butter Energy Bars

Dinner: Roasted Vegetable & Black Bean Tacos

Day: 2

Breakfast: Southwestern Waffle

Drinks: Really Green Smoothie

Lunch: Middle Eastern Savory Yogurt Jar

Snacks: Strawberry-Chocolate Greek Yogurt Bark

Dinner: Spinach & Artichoke Dip Pasta

Day: 3

Breakfast: Egg Salad Avocado Toast

Drinks: Mango & Kale Smoothie

Lunch: Golden Vegetable Soup

Snacks: Peanut Butter Energy Balls

Dinner: Hearty Chickpea & Spinach Stew

Day: 4

Breakfast: Egg Salad Avocado Toast

Drinks: Strawberry-Almond Smoothie

Lunch: Spiced Roasted Cauliflower and Carrots

Snacks: Lemon-Blueberry Bars

Dinner: 20-Minute Balsamic Mushroom & Spinach Pasta

Day: 5

Breakfast: Avocado & Kale Omelet

Drinks: Blueberry & Avocado Smoothie

Lunch: Spinach-Quinoa Bowls With Chicken and Berries

Snacks: Almost Chipotle's Guacamole

Dinner: Kale & Avocado Salad with Blueberries & Edamame

Day: 6

Breakfast: Breakfast Salad with Egg & Salsa Verde Vinaigrette

Drinks: Kale & Pineapple Smoothie

Lunch: Spicy Paleo Veggie Hash

Snacks: Peanut Butter Blueberry Energy Balls

Dinner: One-Pot Lentil & Vegetable Soup with Parmesan

Day: 7

Breakfast: West Coast Avocado Toast

Drinks: Spinach-Avocado Smoothie

Lunch: Turmeric Lamb Chops with Crispy Potatoes and Broccoli

Snacks: Raspberry-Lemon Greek Frozen Yogurt Bark

Dinner: spinach & Artichoke Casserole with Chicken and Cauliflower Rice

Day: 8

Breakfast: Spinach & Feta Scrambled Egg Pitas

Drinks: Kale & Spinach Smoothie

Lunch: Crispy Chicken Thighs with Kale and Chickpeas

Snacks: Roasted Buffalo Chickpeas

Dinner: Quinoa Chili with Sweet Potatoes

Day: 9

Breakfast: Baby Kale Breakfast Salad with Smoked Trout & Avocado

Drinks: Turmeric Latte

Lunch: Lemon-Dill Salmon Pasta Salad

Snacks: Mango-Date Energy Bites

Dinner: One-Pot Lemon-Broccoli Pasta with Parmesan

Day: 10

Breakfast: Avocado & Arugula Omelet

Drinks: Berry Green Smoothie

Lunch: Chickpea-Farro Salad

Snacks: Chickpea Snack Salad

Dinner: Egg Drop Soup with Instant Noodles, Spinach & Scallions

Day: 11

Breakfast: Smoked Trout & Spinach Scrambled Eggs

Drinks: Orange-Mango Gritty with Turmeric and Walnuts

Lunch: Shrimp in Turmeric-Lime Sauce

Snacks: Savory Date & Pistachio Bites

Dinner: Salt & Vinegar Sheet-Pan Chicken & Brussels Sprouts

Day: 12

Breakfast: Mango-Almond Smoothie Bowl

Drinks: Banana-Pineapple-Kale Smoothie

Lunch: Seared Salmon With Zucchini Noodles

Snacks: Vegan Chocolate-Dipped Frozen Banana Bites

Dinner: Salmon & Avocado Poke Bowl

Day: 13

Breakfast: Breakfast Beans with Microwave-Poached Egg

Drinks: Green Tea and Ginger Tonic

Lunch: Spice-Rubbed Chicken with Red Lentil Dal

Snacks: Peanut Butter-Oat Energy Balls

Dinner: Spinach, Lima Bean & Crispy Pancetta Pasta

Day: 14

Breakfast: Avocado & Smoked Salmon Omelet

Drinks: APPLE CARROT BEET SMOOTHIE

Lunch: Air-Fried Cinnamon Apple Chips with Almond Yogurt Dip

Snacks: Homemade Oven-Dried Strawberries

Dinner: Roasted Root Veggies & Greens over Spiced Lentils

Day: 15

Breakfast: Avocado-Egg Toast

Drinks: BEST GREEN JUICE RECIPE

Lunch: Lamb Tagine with Lemon and Olives

Snacks: Peanut Butter-S'mores Greek Yogurt Bark

Dinner: Slow-Cooker Chicken & White Bean Stew

Day: 16

Breakfast: Smoked Salmon Scrambled Eggs

Drinks: BEST TURMERIC SMOOTHIE

Lunch: Kale-and-Chickpea Grain Bowl with Avocado Dressing

Snacks: Air-Fryer Crispy Chickpeas

Dinner: Sheet-Pan Chicken Fajita Bowls

Day: 17

Breakfast: Chia Pudding

Drinks: BLUEBERRY SMOOTHIE

Lunch: Almond-Crusted Trout with Swiss Chard

Snacks: Rice Cake Snackwich

Dinner: Slow-Cooker Mediterranean Diet Stew

Day: 18

Breakfast: Hemp Hearts and Coconut Bar

Drinks: ELDERBERRY TEA

Lunch: This Kale Salad with Spiced Chickpeas and Berries

Snacks: Roasted Beet Hummus

Dinner: Adobo Chicken & Kale Enchiladas

Day: 19

Breakfast: Masala Omelet

Drinks: GINGER SHOTS

Lunch: Chicken and Cucumber Salad With Parsley Pesto

Snacks: Raspberry-Pistachio Greek Yogurt Bark

Dinner: Baked Eggs in Tomato Sauce with Kale

Day: 20

Breakfast: California Breakfast Salad

Drinks: Ginger-Turmeric-Carrot Shots

Lunch: Roasted Salmon with Kale-Quinoa Salad

Snacks: Peanut Butter-Date Energy Balls

Dinner: Mediterranean Chickpea Quinoa Bowl

Day: 21

Breakfast: Granola Breakfast Protein Balls

Drinks: Anti-Inflammatory Golden Tonic

Lunch: Hot Muesli With Pomegranate, Blueberry, and Cashew Crunch

Snacks: Salted Coconut-Caramel Energy Balls

Dinner: Chicken Parmesan & Quinoa Stuffed Peppers

Day: 22

Breakfast: Southwestern Waffle

Drinks: Really Green Smoothie

Lunch: Middle Eastern Savory Yogurt Jar

Snacks: Strawberry-Chocolate Greek Yogurt Bark

Dinner: Spinach & Artichoke Dip Pasta

Day: 23

Breakfast: Egg Salad Avocado Toast

Drinks: Mango & Kale Smoothie

Lunch: Golden Vegetable Soup

Snacks: Peanut Butter Energy Balls

Dinner: Hearty Chickpea & Spinach Stew

Day: 24

Breakfast: Egg Salad Avocado Toast

Drinks: Strawberry-Almond Smoothie

Lunch: Spiced Roasted Cauliflower and Carrots

Snacks: Lemon-Blueberry Bars

Dinner: 20-Minute Balsamic Mushroom & Spinach Pasta

Day: 25

Breakfast: Avocado & Kale Omelet

Drinks: Blueberry & Avocado Smoothie

Lunch: Spinach-Quinoa Bowls With Chicken and Berries

Snacks: Almost Chipotle's Guacamole

Dinner: Kale & Avocado Salad with Blueberries & Edamame

Day: 26

Breakfast: Breakfast Salad with Egg & Salsa Verde Vinaigrette

Drinks: Kale & Pineapple Smoothie

Lunch: Spicy Paleo Veggie Hash

Snacks: Peanut Butter Blueberry Energy Balls

Dinner: One-Pot Lentil & Vegetable Soup with Parmesan

Day: 27

Breakfast: West Coast Avocado Toast

Drinks: Spinach-Avocado Smoothie

Lunch: Turmeric Lamb Chops with Crispy Potatoes and Broccoli

Snacks: Raspberry-Lemon Greek Frozen Yogurt Bark

Dinner: spinach & Artichoke Casserole with Chicken and Cauliflower Rice

Day: 28

Breakfast: Spinach & Feta Scrambled Egg Pitas

Drinks: Kale & Spinach Smoothie

Lunch: Crispy Chicken Thighs with Kale and Chickpeas

Snacks: Roasted Buffalo Chickpeas

Dinner: Quinoa Chili with Sweet Potatoes

Day: 29

Breakfast: Baby Kale Breakfast Salad with Smoked Trout & Avocado

Drinks: Turmeric Latte

Lunch: Lemon-Dill Salmon Pasta Salad

Snacks: Mango-Date Energy Bites

Dinner: One-Pot Lemon-Broccoli Pasta with Parmesan

Day: 30

Breakfast: Avocado & Arugula Omelet

Drinks: Berry Green Smoothie

Lunch: Chickpea-Farro Salad

Snacks: Chickpea Snack Salad

Dinner: Egg Drop Soup with Instant Noodles, Spinach & Scallions

Day: 31

Breakfast: Smoked Trout & Spinach Scrambled Eggs

Drinks: Orange-Mango Gritty with Turmeric and Walnuts

Lunch: Shrimp in Turmeric-Lime Sauce

Snacks: Savory Date & Pistachio Bites

Dinner: Salt & Vinegar Sheet-Pan Chicken & Brussels Sprouts

Chapter 2: Recipes of breakfast

1: Spinach & Egg Scramble with Raspberries

Cook time: 10 min

Total time: 10 min

Servings: 1

Ingredients:

- ½ cup of fresh raspberries
- Pinch of kosher salt
- Pinch of ground pepper
- 2 large eggs, lightly beaten
- 1 teaspoon of canola oil
- 1 slice whole-grain bread, toasted
- 1 ½ cups baby spinach (1 1/2 ounces)

Directions:

- Step 1: A small nonstick skillet should be heated with oil over medium-high heat in step 1. Add the spinach and simmer for 1 to 2 minutes, frequently stirring, until wilted.
- Step 2: Onto a platter, transfer the spinach. Clean the pan, then add eggs and cook it up over medium-low. Cook for 1 to 2 minutes, stirring once or twice to ensure even cooking. Add the salt, spinach, and pepper, and stir.
- Step 3: Along with strawberries and toast, serve the scramble.

Nutrition Facts

Calories: 296, carbohydrates: 20.9g, protein: 17.8g, fat: 4.8g

2: Southwestern Waffle

Cook time: 10 min

Total time: 10 min

Servings: 1

Ingredients:

- 1 egg, cooked sunny-side up
- 1 tablespoon of fresh salsa
- 1 frozen whole-grain waffle, such as Van's 8 Whole Grains Multigrain
- ¼ medium avocado, halved, seeded, peeled and chopped

Directions:

- Step 1:Waffles should be toasted as directed on the packet. Add an avocado, salsa, and egg on top.

Nutrition Facts

Calories: 207, carbohydrates: 17g, protein: 9g, fat: 12g

3: Egg Salad Avocado Toast

Cook time: 5 min

Total time: 5 min

Servings: 1

Ingredients:

- ¼ avocado
- Pinch of salt
- ½ teaspoon juice of lemon
- 1 hard-boiled egg (chopped)
- 1 tablespoon of celery
- ½ teaspoon of hot sauce
- 1 slice whole-wheat toast

Directions:

- Step 1: In a small bowl, mash avocado with spicy sauce, lemon juice, celery, and salt. Add the egg (hard-boiled) and combine. Apply to toast.

Nutrition Facts

Calories: 230, carbohydrates: 17.2g, protein: 10.9g, fat: 13.7g

4: Smoked Salmon & Cream Cheese Omelet

Cook time: 10 min

Total time: 15 min

Servings: 1

Ingredients:

- 2 large eggs
- 1 teaspoon butter
- Pinch of salt
- 2 tablespoons chopped smoked salmon
- 1 teaspoon of reduced-fat milk or water
- 1 tablespoon of red onion (finely chopped)
- ⅛ teaspoon of ground pepper (plus more for garnish)
- 1 tablespoon of cream cheese, softened, or crumbled feta
- 1 ½ teaspoon of chopped fresh dill, plus more for garnish

Directions:

- Step 1: In a small bowl, whisk together the eggs, milk (or water), pepper, and salt.
- Step 2: In a small nonstick skillet over low heat, melt the butter, swirling the pan to ensure that the entire bottom is covered. Add the egg mixture and heat it without stirring for one minute.
- Step 3: Over one-half eggs, top with cheese, salmon, dill, and onion. For one minute, cook. Lift the exposed side of the pan with a flexible spatula to allow the raw egg from the centre to flow below; you might need to slightly tilt the pan. Lift the mixture in various locations until there is hardly any raw egg remaining on top. 2 more minutes of cooking.
- Step 4: Flip the bare side of the omelette over the filling with the spatula, fold it in half, and cook for one minute. (Lower the heat if eggs are beginning to brown.) After carefully turning it over, heat it for another minute. Serve right now and top with additional pepper and dill, if desired.

Nutrition Facts

Calories: 254, carbohydrates: 2.7g, protein: 16.8g, fat: 19.2g

5: Avocado & Kale Omelet

Cook time: 10 min

Total time: 10 min

Servings: 1

Ingredients:

- 2 large eggs
- 1 cup of chopped kale
- 1 teaspoon of unsalted sunflower seeds
- Pinch of crushed red pepper
- 1 tablespoon of lime juice
- Pinch of salt
- 1 teaspoon of milk (low-fat)
- 1 tablespoon of cilantro (chopped fresh)
- ¼ avocado, sliced
- 2 teaspoons of olive oil (extra-virgin)

Directions:

- Step 1: In small bowl, whisk together the eggs, salt, and milk. In small skillet (nonstick) over medium heat, warm 1 teaspoon of oil.
- Step 2: Add the egg mixture and cook for 1 to 2 minutes, or until the bottom is set, but the middle is still a little runny. After about 35 seconds, flip the omelette over and cook it until it is set. Place on a platter.
- Step 3: Combine the lime juice, remaining one teaspoon of oil, cilantro, red pepper (crushed), and the kale with all these ingredients. Add the kale and avocado salad to the omelette as garnish.

Nutrition Facts

Calories: 339, carbohydrates: 8.6g, protein: 15g, fat: 28.1g

6: Breakfast Salad with Egg & Salsa Verde Vinaigrette

Cook time: 10 min

Total time: 10 min

Servings: 1

Ingredients:

- 1 large egg
- 2 cups of salad greens or mesclun
- ½ cup canned of beans (red kidney)
- ¼ of avocado, sliced
- 1 tablespoon plus 1 tsp. of olive oil (extra-virgin)
- 8 blue corn tortilla chips, broken into large pieces
- 2 tablespoons of chopped cilantro (plus more for garnish)
- 3 tablespoons of salsa verde, such as Frontera brand

Directions:

- Step 1: In small bowl, combine the salsa, one tbsp. Of oil, and the cilantro. Place half of the mixture in the shallow bowl of dinner with the mesclun (or other greens).
- Step 2: Arrange avocado, beans, and chips on top of salad.
- Step 3: In small skillet (nonstick) over the medium-high flame, warm the final teaspoon of oil. Add the egg and cook for about two minutes, or until white is fully cooked but yolk is still a little runny.
- Step 4: Arrange the salad with egg. Add more cilantro, if desired, and drizzle with the leftover the salsa vinaigrette.

Nutrition Facts:

Calories: 527, carbohydrates: 37g, protein: 16g, fat: 34g

7: West Coast Avocado Toast

Cook time: 10 min

Total time: 10 min

Servings: 1

Ingredients:

- 1 teaspoon of vinegar (red wine)
- Pinch of pepper
- ¼ cup of alfalfa sprouts
- Pinch of salt
- ¼ avocado, sliced
- ¼ cup of plain hummus
- 1 cup of salad greens (mixed)
- 1 teaspoon of olive oil (extra-virgin)
- 2 slices of sprouted whole-wheat bread, toasted
- 2 teaspoons of sunflower seeds (unsalted)

Directions:

- Step 1: In a medium bowl, combine greens with oil, pepper, salt, and the vinegar. Each piece of toast is spread with two tablespoons of hummus.
- Step 2: Sprinkle sunflower seeds on top and add sprouts, avocado, and greens.

Nutrition Facts

Calories: 429, carbohydrates: 46.4g, protein: 16.2g, fat: 21.9g

8: Spinach & Feta Egg Pitas of Scrambled

Cook time: 15 min

Total time: 15 min

Servings: 4

Ingredients:

- 8 eggs, beaten
- Pinch salt
- Pepper to taste (Freshly ground)
- 1 tablespoon of olive oil (extra-virgin)
- 8 teaspoons of sun-dried tomato (tapenade or pesto)
- ¼ cup of crumbled feta cheese
- 1 (10 ounces) block frozen chopped spinach, thawed, drained and squeezed dry
- 4 whole-wheat of pitas, cut in half

Directions:

- Step 1: Place large skillet (nonstick) over the medium heat and add oil. While stirring occasionally, boil the salt and spinach until it is steaming hot.
- Step 2: Add the eggs and simmer, turning eggs as they set, for 4 to 5 minutes, or until form soft curds and the barely moist. Cook the pepper and feta until it has set.
- Step 3: Spread 2 tbsp. of tapenade (or pesto) into each pita pocket. Among the pitas, distribute egg mixture.

Nutrition Facts

Calories: 303, carbohydrates: 21.1g, protein: 19.9g, fat: 16.2g

9: Baby Kale Breakfast Salad with Smoked Trout & Avocado

Cook time: 0 min

Total time: 15 min

Servings: 1

Ingredients:

- Pinch of salt
- Pinch of pepper
- 2 teaspoons of vinegar (red wine)
- ¼ cup of smoked trout (flaked)
- 1 teaspoon of minced garlic
- ¼ firm ripe avocado, sliced or diced
- 3 cups of baby kale (lightly packed)
- 1 tablespoon of olive oil (extra-virgin)
- 1 tablespoon of red onion (finely chopped)

Directions:

- Step 1: Use the side of a chef's knife to mash the garlic and the salt into a paste. In one medium-sized bowl, combine the garlic paste, vinegar, oil, and pepper.
- Step 2: Kale is added in Step 2 and coated. Serve with red onion, avocado, and fish on top.

Nutrition Facts:

Calories: 275, carbohydrates: 9.4g, protein: 10.1g, fat: 23g

10: Avocado & Arugula Omelet

Cook time: 10 min

Total time: 10 min

Servings: 1

Ingredients:

- 2 large eggs
- 1/8 teaspoon of salt, divided
- 1 teaspoon juice of lemon
- 1/2 cup arugula
- 1 teaspoon of milk (low-fat)
- 1/4 avocado, diced
- 2 teaspoons of olive oil (extra-virgin)
- 2 tablespoons of Greek yoghurt (plain whole milk)

Directions:

- Step 1: In a small bowl, whisk together the eggs, milk, and a touch of salt. In a small skillet (nonstick) over the medium heat, warm one teaspoon of oil.
- Step 2: Add egg mixture and cook for 2 minutes, or until the bottom is set but the middle is still a little runny. After 30 seconds, flip the omelette over and cook it until it is set. Place on a platter.
- Step 3: Combine the arugula in a small bowl with the remaining one teaspoon oil and the lemon juice. Arugula, yoghurt, avocado, and final pinch of the salt are sprinkled on top of the omelette.

Nutrition Facts:

Calories: 344, carbohydrates: 7.2g, protein: 16.9g, fat: 28g

11: Smoked Trout & Spinach Scrambled Eggs

Cook time: 15 min

Total time: 15 min

Servings: 2

Ingredients:

- ¼ teaspoon of ground pepper
- 2 tablespoons of shallot (finely chopped)
- Pinch of salt
- 4 large eggs
- 1 cup of spinach (chopped)
- 2 tablespoons of milk (reduced-fat)
- 2 teaspoons of grapeseed oil or avocado oil
- ½ cup of boned and flaked smoked trout

Directions:

- Step 1: Whisk the milk, eggs, salt, and pepper in a medium bowl until the mixture is evenly light yellow in color.
- Step 2: Heat the oil over medium heat in a medium nonstick skillet. When the shallot has started to turn color, add it and stir for 1 to 2 minutes. The egg mixture is then added, and medium or low heat is then used. Cook, occasionally stirring, for 30 seconds or until the edges start to set.
- Step 3: Put the trout on top of the eggs in step three. Use a rubber spatula to gently push and fold beat eggs until they are barely set and foamy about 4 minutes. Spinach is added; stir. In order for the spinach to barely wilt, remove from the heat, cover, and let stand for 2 minutes.

Nutrition Facts

243 calories; protein 19g; carbohydrates 3.9g; fat 16.7g

12: Mango-Almond Smoothie Bowl

Cook time: 10 min

Total time: 10 min

Servings: 1

Ingredients:

- ⅛ teaspoon of ground allspice
- ¼ cup of raspberries
- ¼ cup of banana (frozen sliced)
- ½ teaspoon of honey
- ½ cup of chopped mango (frozen)
- ¼ cup of almond milk (plain unsweetened)
- ½ cup of yoghurt (nonfat plain Greek)
- 5 tablespoons of unsalted almonds, divided

Directions:

- Step 1: The first step is to thoroughly combine the almond milk, yoghurt, mango, banana, allspice, and 3 tablespoons of almonds in blender.
- Step 2: Transfer the smoothie to a bowl, then garnish with raspberries and with the remaining two tablespoons of almonds and the honey.

Nutrition Facts

Calories: 457, carbohydrates: 45.8g, protein: 21.6g, fat: 24.1g

13: Breakfast Beans with Microwave-Poached Egg

Cook time: 15 min

Total time: 15 min

Servings: 2

Ingredients:

- ½ cup of cooked barley
- 1 cup of water, divided
- ⅛ teaspoon of salt
- 2 teaspoons of canola oil
- 2 large eggs, divided

- ½ teaspoon of ground cumin
- ⅛ teaspoon of hot sauce
- ½ avocado, sliced
- ¼ cup of red bell pepper (chopped)
- 2 tablespoons of pepper Jack cheese (shredded)
- 1 teaspoon of white vinegar (distilled)
- ¾ cup of rinsed canned black beans (low-sodium)
- 2 tablespoons of coarse cilantro (chopped fresh)
- 2 chopped scallions, whites and greens separated
- ½ cup low-sodium chicken broth or vegetable broth

Directions:

- Step 1: In the first step, warm the oil in a medium skillet over medium heat. Add scallion whites, cumin, and bell pepper; simmer for 2 minutes, frequently stirring, until softened.
- Step 2: Include the cooked barley, beans, salt, and broth. Cook for 3 to 5 minutes or until most of the liquid has been absorbed. Add spicy sauce and scallion greens after mixing. Divide between 2 bowls.
- Step 3: Mix half cup of water and 1/2 teaspoon of vinegar in a small bowl that can go in the microwave. One egg should be carefully cracked into the water and soaked completely. For about a minute on High, covered with a microwave-safe plate, microwave the egg until the white is set, but the yolk is still a little runny. (Continue to microwave if required, checking every 10 seconds.)
- Step 4: Place the egg on top of the bean mixture in one bowl after removing it with a slotted spoon and drying it off. Repeat with the remaining egg, 1/2 teaspoon. Vinegar, and ½ cup water.
- Step 5: Add 1 Tbsp. Cheese and ¼ avocado to each bowl. If preferred, add cilantro to the dish.

Nutrition Facts

Calories: 364, carbohydrates: 32g, protein: 16g, fat: 20g

14: Avocado & Smoked Salmon Omelet

Cook time: 10 min

Total time: 10 min

Servings: 1

Ingredients

- 2 large eggs
- Pinch of salt
- 1 ounce of smoked salmon
- 1 teaspoon of milk (low-fat)
- ¼ avocado, sliced
- 1 tablespoon of fresh basil (chopped)
- 1 teaspoon of olive oil plus 1/2 teaspoon (extra-virgin)

Directions

- Step 1: In a small bowl, whisk together the eggs, milk, and salt. In a small nonstick skillet over medium heat, warm 1 teaspoon of oil.
- Step 2: Add egg mixture and cook for 1 to 2 minutes, or until the bottom is set but the middle is still a little runny. After 30 seconds, flip up omelette over and then cook it until it is set. Place it on platter.
- Step 3: Add salmon, avocado, and basil over top. Add the final 1/2 tsp. of oil in a drizzle.

Nutrition Facts

Calories: 323, carbohydrates: 5.3g, protein: 19g, fat: 252g

15: Avocado-Egg Toast

Cook time: 5 min

Total time: 5 min

Servings: 1

Ingredients

- ¼ avocado
- 1 large egg, fried
- 1 teaspoon of Sriracha (Optional)

- ¼ teaspoon of ground pepper
- 1 slice of whole-wheat bread, toasted
- ⅛ teaspoon of garlic powder
- 1 tablespoon of scallion, sliced (Optional)

Directions

- Step 1: Gently mash the avocado after adding the garlic powder and pepper to the small bowl.
- Step 2: Add the mixture of avocado and the fried egg to the toast. If desired, garnish with scallion and Sriracha.

Nutrition Facts

Calories: 271, carbohydrates: 18.1g, protein: 11.5g, fat: 17.7g

Chapter 3: Recipes of lunch:

1: Caprese Snack Skewers

Cook time: 0 min

Total time: 3 min

Servings: 1

Ingredients

- 6 cherry tomato
- 6 balls of Ciliegine Mozzarella (Whole Milk)
- 6 Basil Leaves

Directions

- Step 1: Thread two (8-inch) bamboo skewers with ciliegine mozzarella, cherry tomatoes, and basil leaves (mozzarella balls the size of cherry tomatoes).
- Step 2: Serving at room temperature is step two.

Nutrition Facts

Calories: 150, carbohydrates: 4g, protein: 13g, fat: 9g

2: Middle Eastern Savory Yogurt Jar

Cook time: 0 min

Total time: 3 min

Servings: 1

Ingredients

- 2 cups of Greek Yogurt (Plain Nonfat)
- 1 oz Chipotle Crunchy Chickpeas
- 1/4 tsp sea salt
- 1/4 cup of Cheese (Crumbled Feta)
- 2 tbsp of olive oil (extra-virgin)
- 1 tbsp of mint leaves (fresh)
- 1/4 tsp of black pepper (ground)
- 2 Wedge of lemon Juice, Raw

Directions

- Step 1: Fill two containers or bowls with yoghurt that have a capacity of 10 ounces.
- Step 2: Top with feta cheese, salt, pepper, olive oil, and crispy chickpeas. (Tip: Toasted pine nuts and a sprinkle of the cayenne pepper can be used as a substitute for spicy, crispy chickpeas.)
- Step 3: If using, garnish with the mint and serve with lemon wedges.

Nutrition Facts

Calories: 334, carbohydrates: 17g, protein: 27g, fat: 18g

3: Golden Vegetable Soup

Cook time: 30 min

Total time: 40 min

Servings: 4

Ingredients

- 1 white onion, chopped
- 1-inch ginger, peeled and minced
- 1/2 teaspoon of ground cumin
- 1/8 teaspoon of cayenne pepper (optional)
- 32 ounces of chicken bone broth
- 1 cup of sweet potato chunks (frozen)
- 2 tablespoons of lemon juice
- 1 teaspoon of olive oil (extra virgin)
- 1green apple, peeled and chopped
- 1/4 cup of plain yoghurt (nonfat)
- 2 cloves garlic, minced
- 1/2 teaspoon of ground turmeric
- 1 tablespoon of green onions (chopped)
- 2 organic carrots, scrubbed clean and chopped

Directions

- Step 1: Heat olive oil over medium-low heat in a sizable, heavy-bottomed pot. Saute onions until they are transparent and tender.
- Step 2: Add the ginger and garlic; sauté for about 30 seconds, or until aromatic and golden. Stir in the cayenne (optional), cumin, and turmeric.
- Step 3: Add chunks of potato, apple, and carrot to the saucepan. Add bone broth on top, then boil the dish. Cook for 25–30 minutes, or until soft, covered.
- Step 4: Puree the soup using a countertop or immersion blender until it is smooth. Divide into bowls after adding lemon juice.
- Step 5: Add yoghurt and sprinkle onions over top. If desired, add extra cayenne to the dust.

Nutrition Facts

Calories: 147, carbohydrates: 27g, protein: 7g, fat: 2.8g

4: Spiced Roasted Cauliflower and Carrots

Cook time: 10 min

Total time: 25 min

Servings: 2

Ingredients

- 2 cups of sliced carrot (thinly diagonally)
- 3 tablespoons olive oil
- 1/4 teaspoon of black pepper
- 3/4 teaspoon of ground cumin
- 3/8 teaspoon of kosher salt
- 1/4 cup of pomegranate arils
- 3 cups of cauliflower florets
- 1/2 teaspoon of ground cinnamon
- 2 tablespoons fresh cilantro (chopped)

Directions

- Step 1: First, turn the broiler to high. In a big basin, mix the cumin, carrot, cinnamon, pepper, and salt with the cauliflower florets.
- Step 2: Spread on a baking sheet lined with foil in step two. 8 to 10 minutes in the broiler, stirring once every 4 minutes. Add some cilantro and pomegranate seeds on top.

Nutrition Facts

Calories: 154, carbohydrates: 13g, protein: 2g, fat: 11g

5: Spinach-Quinoa Bowls With Chicken and Berries

Cook time: 0 min

Total time: 35 min

Servings: 2

Ingredients

- 1 cup of cooked quinoa
- 2 tablespoons of cheese (crumbled feta)
- 1 tablespoon of sliced almonds, toasted

- 1 tablespoon of vinegar (white wine)
- 2/3 cup of chicken breast (chopped cooked)
- 1/4 teaspoon of Dijon mustard
- 2 tablespoons of olive oil (extra-virgin)
- 1/2 teaspoon of honey
- 3 cups of baby spinach or mixed greens
- 2 tablespoons of cheese (crumbled feta)
- 1/2 teaspoon of kosher salt
- 1/2 cup of blueberries or sliced strawberries

Directions

- Step 1: Distribute the chicken, spinach, and quinoa equally among two 1-quart sealed containers. Cheese, berries, and the almonds should be distributed evenly over each salad until you are ready to serve, cover and chill.
- Step 2: Combine the mustard, oil, honey, vinegar, and the salt in a small bowl just before serving. Serve the salads right away after evenly distributing the dressing among them and tossing them to combine.
- Step 3: Dairy-Free Alternative: Leave off the feta cheese and up the amount of almond slices to 3 tablespoons.

Nutrition Facts

Calories: 396, carbohydrates: 31g, protein: 23g, fat: 20g

6: Spicy Paleo Veggie Hash

Cook time: 12 min

Total time: 35 min

Servings: 3

Ingredients

- 2 tablespoons olive oil
- 2 tablespoons fresh oregano (chopped)
- 3/4 teaspoon of kosher salt, divided
- 1/4 cup pumpkinseed kernels (unsalted)

- 1/2 teaspoon of ground cumin
- 5 garlic cloves, minced
- 1/2 teaspoon of ground cinnamon
- 1 plum tomato, seeded and diced
- 1/4 teaspoon of red pepper (ground)
- 1 1/4 cups of water, divided
- 3 cups sweet potato (diced peeled)
- 1 cup green beans, trimmed and cut into 1-inch

Directions

- Step 1: In the first step, a sizable pan is heated over medium-high heat. Spatula with oil added; stir. Potato, oregano, and 1/2 teaspoon salt should be added. Cook for 3 minutes while stirring occasionally.
- Step 2: Cook for a minute after adding the cumin, cinnamon, red pepper, and garlic. Adding 1/2 cup of water, cover, and cook for 5 minutes on low heat. Cook for two minutes after taking off the cover. Pan from the heat.
- Step 3: In a saucepan, bring the remaining 3/4 cup water to a boil. Cook the green beans for 4 minutes after adding the final 1/4 teaspoon of salt.
- Step 4: Distribute the potato mixture evenly among the four shallow bowls, and top each with one tablespoon tomato and one tablespoon pumpkin seeds.

Nutrition Facts

Calories: 209, carbohydrates: 25g, protein: 5g, fat: 10.8g

7: Turmeric Lamb Chops with Crispy Potatoes and Broccoli

Cook time: 13 min

Total time: 20 min

Servings: 3

Ingredients

- 1 tablespoon of water
- 3 tablespoons of olive oil, divided
- 1 1/4 teaspoons of kosher salt, divided
- 2 teaspoons of ground cumin
- 8 (3-oz.) lamb loin chops
- 1 teaspoon of ground turmeric
- 1 tablespoon of unsalted butter, softened
- 1/2 teaspoon of black pepper, divided
- 1 (12-oz.) pkg. broccoli florets (fresh steam-in-bag)
- 1 lemon, cut into wedges
- 12 ounces baby Yukon Gold potatoes, quartered (about 2 1/2 cups)

Directions

- Step 1: In a medium microwave-safe bowl, add 1 tablespoon water and the potatoes. Wrap the bowl in plastic.
- Step 2: Heat for 4 minutes on high or until tender. Potatoes should be spread out in a single layer and dried for three minutes on a baking sheet lined with paper towels.
- Step 3: Combine 1 tablespoon oil, 1 teaspoon each of cumin, turmeric, salt, and pepper in a small bowl. Sprinkle lamb chops with the spice mixture equally.
- Step 4: In a big cast-iron skillet over medium-high heat, add 1 tablespoon of oil. Add the lamb chops to the pan and cook for three minutes on each side for medium-rare or to the desired doneness. Remove chops from pan; let stand for 5 minutes.

- Step 5: Reset the pan to medium-high. The last tablespoon of oil. Add the potatoes, the remaining 1/2 tsp. of pepper, and ½ teaspoon of salt. Cook for 4 minutes, or until the potatoes are crisp.
- Step 6: Prepare broccoli per the instructions on the package. In a bowl, combine the broccoli, butter, and remaining 1/4 tsp. Salt. Toss to combine. Lemon wedges, lamb, and potato mixture should be served with.

Nutrition Facts

Calories: 453, carbohydrates: 22g, protein: 40g, fat: 24g

8: Crispy Chicken Thighs with Kale and Chickpeas

Cook time: 43 min

Total time: 43 min

Servings: 4

Ingredients

- 2 teaspoons of olive oil
- 1 teaspoon of ground coriander
- Half teaspoon of black pepper
- 1 red (vertically sliced)
- 3/4 teaspoon of salt (kosher)
- 4 cloves of garlic (sliced)
- 8 ounces of stemmed (torn curly of kale)
- 4 skin-on, bone-in chicken thighs, patted dry with paper towels
- 1 can of chickpeas (drained and rinsed)

Directions

- Step 1: Turn on the oven up to 450 Fahrenheit.
- Step 2: Sprinkle both of the sides of the chicken with a mixture of coriander, half tsp. of salt, and quarter tsp. pepper. A sizable cast-iron pan or another ovenproof skillet should be heated to medium.
- Step 3: Add the oil and stir the pan to coat. Skin-side down, put the chicken to the pan. Cook the chicken for eight minutes or till the skin is just beginning to brown.
- Step 4: Add the remaining quarter tsp. each of pepper and salt to the drippings in the pan and heat for three minutes or till the onion is tender. Add the first half of the kale; cook and cover for two min, or until just wilted. The remaining kale is added, stirred, and covered. Cook for two min, or until just wilted. Stir.
- Step 5: Place the chicken, the side of skin will be up, on top of the chickpeas. Bake chicken uncovered at the 450°F for ten to twelve minutes, or until an internal thermometer reads 165°F.

Nutrition Facts

Calories: 440, carbohydrates: 27g, protein: 47g, fat: 18g

9: Lemon-Dill Salmon Pasta Salad

Cook time: 43 min

Total time: 43 min

Servings: 4

Ingredients

- 1 teaspoon zest of lemon
- 1/2 teaspoon of salt (kosher)
- 1/4 tsp. of black pepper
- 1 cup of cucumber (thinly sliced)
- 2 1/2 tablespoons juice of lemon
- 1 cup of peas (thawed, frozen)
- 1/3 cup red onion (thinly sliced)
- 2 (6-oz.) cans of wild sockeye salmon (drained, skinless, boneless)
- 2 tablespoons of olive oil (extra-virgin)
- 8 ounces of chickpea rotini, shells, or penne
- 3 tablespoons of chopped dill

Directions

- Step 1: Prepare the pasta as directed on the package, removing the fat and salt. Drain completely, then thoroughly rinse with ice-cold water.
- Step 2: In a sizable bowl, whisk together the oil, salt, pepper, lemon zest, and lemon juice.
- Step 3: Put the onion in the colander or strainer and wash it under cold water. Good drainage
- Step 4: Toss the cucumber, pasta, salmon, onion, peas, and dill with the vinaigrette.

Nutrition Facts

Calories: 436, carbohydrates: 43g, protein: 36g, fat: 15g

10: Chickpea-Farro Salad

Cook time: 0 min

Total time: 43 min

Servings: 4

Ingredients

- 2 tablespoons of olive oil (extra-virgin)
- 1/2 cup of diced celery
- 1/2 teaspoon of kosher salt
- 1/4 teaspoon of black pepper (freshly ground)
- 1 tablespoon of vinegar (red wine)
- 1 cup faro (cooked)
- 2 tablespoons of minced shallots
- 1 cup canned of chickpeas, rinsed and drained
- 1/2 cup celery leaves (coarsely chopped)

Directions

- Step 1: Using a whisk, combine the first five ingredients in large bowl. Then, combine the remaining ingredients and coat.

Nutrition Facts

Calories: 171, carbohydrates: 21g, protein: 4g, fat: 8g

11: Shrimp in Turmeric-Lime Sauce

Cook time: 7 min

Total time: 35 min

Servings: 4

Ingredients

- 1 tablespoon of olive oil
- 1 tablespoon of lime zest
- 2 teaspoons of fish sauce
- 2 teaspoons of chilli sauce (sriracha)
- 4 cloves garlic, minced

- 2 1/2 tablespoons of butter
- 1 tablespoon of ground turmeric
- 1/2 cup Cilantro Leaves (Fresh)
- 3 tablespoons juice of lime
- 1/2 teaspoon of black pepper (freshly ground)
- 3 tablespoons of green onions(thinly sliced)
- 1/2 teaspoon of black pepper (freshly ground)

Directions

- Step 1: Cook shrimp for 30 seconds or just until they are opaque in a large saucepan of salted boiling water. Place on a baking sheet covered with paper towels and let drain.
- Step 2: In a bowl, combine the lime zest, oil, lime juice, garlic, turmeric, sriracha, fish sauce, and pepper. Whisk to combine. Set apart.
- Step 3: In the third step, melt butter in a big skillet over medium heat. Once the sauce has become fragrant, add the turmeric-lime sauce.
- Step 4: Add the shrimp and cook, gently stirring and adjusting heat as necessary to maintain sauce just below a simmer, for about 5 minutes, or until shrimp is cooked through.
- Step 5: Add cilantro and green onions as garnish in step 5.

Nutrition Facts

Calories: 192, carbohydrates: 5g, protein: 16g, fat: 12g

12: Seared Salmon with Zucchini Noodles

Cook time: 10 min

Total time: 15 min

Servings: 1

Ingredients

- 1/2 teaspoon of olive oil
- 1 cup of spiralized zucchini (from 1 large zucchini)
- 1/8 teaspoon of kosher salt
- 1/4 cup of carrot ribbons (from 1 medium carrot)
- 1/8 teaspoon of black pepper
- 6 ounces of salmon fillet (skin-on wild-caught)
- 2 tablespoons of Avocado-Herb Dressing

Directions

- Step 1: First, evenly distribute the salt and pepper over the salmon. A medium nonstick skillet is warmed up. For about 6 minutes, cook the salmon with the skin side down.
- Step 2: Drizzle some oil over the salmon, flip it over, and cook for another three minutes, or until it's cooked to your liking. Toss onto a platter.
- Step 3: Add the zucchini and carrot to the skillet and stir continually for 1 minute, or until they are just heated through.
- Step 4: Transfer to a bowl and add the salmon on top. Apply a dressing drizzle. Serve instantly.

Nutrition Facts

Calories: 430, carbohydrates: 10g, protein: 36g, fat: 27g

13: Spice-Rubbed Chicken with Red Lentil Dal

Cook time: 45 min

Total time: 1 hr. 5 min

Servings: 4

Ingredients

- 1 cup of onion (finely chopped)
- 3 cups of water
- 2 tablespoons of canola oil, divided
- 5 ounces of baby spinach (fresh)
- 1 1/2 teaspoons of ground turmeric, divided
- 3/4 teaspoon of ground cumin
- 3 garlic cloves, minced
- 1/2 teaspoon of ground coriander
- 1 cup of red lentils (dried)
- 1/2 teaspoon of black pepper (freshly ground)
- 1/4 teaspoon of red pepper (ground)
- 1/4 teaspoon of ginger(dried ground)
- 2 bay leaves (dried)
- 4 (4-oz.) skinless, boneless chicken thighs
- 7/8 teaspoon of kosher salt, divided
- 1 cup cherry tomatoes (halved)

Directions

- Step 1: First, set a sizable pot on a medium heat. Swirl in 1 1/2 tablespoons of oil to coat. With occasional stirring, sauté the onion for three minutes. Cook the garlic for 2 minutes while stirring constantly.
- Step 2: Stir continuously while cooking 1 teaspoon each of red pepper and turmeric for 30 seconds. Stir in the bay leaves, water, and lentils before bringing them to a boil. Simmer for about 25 minutes, reducing heat as necessary, until thick and creamy.
- Step 3: Throw away the bay leaves. Add salt, 1/2 teaspoon plus 1/8 teaspoon, and stir. Add the spinach little by little while stirring it to wilt.

- Step 4: Concoct a mixture of the remaining 1/2 teaspoon turmeric, 1/4 teaspoon salt, cumin, coriander, black pepper, and ginger in the meantime.
- Step 5: Distribute evenly over the top and bottom of the chicken thighs. Over medium-high heat, preheat a large skillet.
- Step 6: Add the final 1 1/2 teaspoons of oil and stir to combine in step 6. Cook the chicken in the pan for five minutes on each side or until done.
- Step 7: Combined with tomatoes and lentil dal, serve chicken.

Nutrition Facts

Calories: 403, carbohydrates: 36g, protein: 38g, fat: 12g

14: Air-Fried Cinnamon Apple Chips With Almond Yogurt Dip

Cook time: 35 min

Total time: 35 min

Servings: 4

Ingredients

- 1 teaspoon of ground cinnamon
- Cooking spray
- 1/4 cup Greek yoghurt (plain 1% low-fat)
- 2 teaspoons of canola oil
- 1 tablespoon of almond butter
- 1 (8-oz.) apple (such as Honeycrisp or Fuji)
- 1 teaspoon of honey

Directions

- Step 1: On a mandoline, slice an apple thinly in step 1. Slices should be combined with oil and cinnamon in a basin. Stir to combine.
- Step 2: Spray the air fryer basket with cooking spray thoroughly. Cook at 375°F for 12 minutes, flipping the slices every 4 minutes and rearranging them to flatten them since they will move during the cooking process. Place 7 to 8 apple slices in a single layer in the basket.
- Step 3: Slices won't be entirely crisped, but they'll keep getting crispier as they cool. Repeat with the rest of the apple pieces.

- Step 4: Blend the yoghurt, almond butter, and honey in a small bowl while the apple slices cook. Place 6 to 8 apple slices and a small dollop of dipping sauce on each plate before serving.

Nutrition Facts

Calories: 104, carbohydrates: 17g, protein: 2g, fat: 3g

15: Lamb Tagine With Lemon and Olives

Cook Time: 2 hrs.

Total Time: 2 hrs. 45 min

Servings: 6

Ingredients

- 2 pounds boneless leg of lamb, trimmed
- 1 tablespoon of olive oil, divided
- 1 tablespoon of fresh ginger (minced peeled)
- 1/2 teaspoon of ground cinnamon
- 1/4 teaspoon red pepper (divided, ground)
- 3 garlic cloves, minced
- 3 cups of chicken stock (unsalted)
- 1 cup of yellow onion (chopped)
- 3/4 teaspoon of kosher salt, divided
- 18 pitted green olives (rinsed, drained, and halved)
- 1 teaspoon of cumin (ground roasted)
- 1/4 cup of fresh cilantro (chopped)
- 1/2 cup of golden raisins
- 3 tablespoons of juice of lemon
- 1/8 teaspoon of saffron threads (crushed)
- 3 cups of Israeli couscous (hot cooked)
- 4 medium carrots, peeled and cut diagonally into 1-in. pieces

Directions

- Step 1: First, season the lamb with 1/2 tsp. Salt and 1/8 tsp. Red pepper. A sizable Dutch oven is warmed at medium-high. Add two teaspoons of oil and stir to coat the pan. Stir in half the meat, cooking for 5 minutes or until browned. Get the lamb out of the skillet and place it on a platter. Repeat with the other lamb.

- Step 2: Fill the pan with 1 teaspoon of oil. 2 minutes of sautéing includes the addition of 1/8 teaspoon red pepper, onion, ginger, cumin, cinnamon, saffron, and garlic. Lamb, any accumulated juices, and stock are added; the mixture is simmered.
- Step 3: Cook for 15 minutes with the lid on and the heat reduced to medium. Add the carrot and a dash of salt, stirring. Cover partially and cook for one hour. Include the raisins and olives. Add cilantro and juice after removing from heat. Serve alongside couscous.

Nutrition Facts

Calories: 421, carbohydrates: 38g, protein: 37g, fat: 13g

16: Ginger-Lime Fruit Salad

Cook time: 0 min

Total time: 5 min

Servings: 6

Ingredients

- Half cup of blueberries
- 1 teaspoon of lime rind (grated)
- 1 cup of ripe mango (chopped)
- 1 tablespoon juice of lime
- 1 cup of quartered strawberries
- 1/2 teaspoon of grated ginger

Directions

- Step 1: In one bowl, combine all the ingredients; let stand for Five minutes before eating.

Nutrition Facts

Calories: 49, carbohydrates: 12g, protein: 1g, fat: 0.3g

17: Chickpea grain and kale bowl with the Avocado Dressing

Cook time: 20 min

Total time: 40 min

Servings: 6

Ingredients

- One and half tablespoons of canola oil
- 1 tablespoon juice of lemon
- 4 cups of lacinato kale (chopped)
- Half cup of shallots (vertically sliced)
- 3/4 tsp. of divided kosher salt
- 1 cup of boiling water
- Half teaspoon of black pepper
- Half cup of uncooked bulgur
- 2 tablespoons of olive oil (extra-virgin)
- 1 tablespoon of water
- 2 cups of chopped carrots
- 1 tbsp. tahini paste well stirred (sesame seed)
- Half cup of parsley leaves (fresh flat-leaf)
- one garlic clove
- Half avocado, pitted and peeled
- 1/4 tsp. ground turmeric
- 2 chickpeas cans unsalted, rinsed and drained

Directions

- Step 1: In the first step, place bulgur in one medium dish with 1 cup of boiling water. Wait 10 minutes, then thoroughly drain.
- Step 2: Use paper towels to pat the chickpeas dry. A big skillet with canola oil over high heat. Add the carrots and chickpeas; simmer, stirring periodically, for about 6 minutes, or until the chickpeas are nicely browned.
- Step 3: Add the kale; cover the pan, and cook for 2 minutes, or until the carrots are soft. Toss in the shallots, half teaspoon of salt, parsley, and the chickpea mixture along as the bulgur.

- Step 4: Avocado, one tablespoon of water, olive oil, tahini, garlic, juice, turmeric, and the last one fourth teaspoon of salt are all blended together in the food processor till it is smooth. Toss the avocado mixture evenly over the bulgur mixture in each of the four bowls.

Nutrition Facts

Calories: 520, carbohydrates: 68g, protein: 18g, fat: 20g

18: Swiss Chard with Trout (Almond-Crusted)

Cook Time: 25 min

Total time: 40 min

Servings: 4

Ingredients

- 4 (4- to 5-oz.) skin-on trout fillets
- 1 tablespoon of Dijon mustard
- 4 lemon wedges
- Half teaspoon divided black pepper
- 3 thinly sliced garlic cloves
- 1 tbsp. lemon juice (fresh)
- 3/4 teaspoon kosher salt, divided
- 1/4 cup white wine (dry)
- 1 3/4 ounces almond flour (about half cup)
- 1 tbsp. unsalted butter
- 2 1/2 tablespoons grapeseed or canola oil, divided
- 1 tablespoon fresh chives (minced)
- 4 cups thinly sliced Swiss chard leaves and stems (about 5 3/8 oz.)

Directions

- Step 1: First, put the almond flour into the small basin. The skin side of the fish fillets should remain uncovered while you lightly push the side of the each fillet which is mustard into the almond flour.
- Step 2: In step two, a sizable nonstick pan is heated to medium-high heat with 1 tablespoon of oil. Flesh it side down, add 2 fillets and heat for two to three minutes, or until golden brown and somewhat crispy. The flesh should be flaky and well-cooked thoroughly after turning the fillets. Put on a plate that has been covered with the paper towels.
- Step 3: After cleaning the skillet, repeat steps 2 and 3 using the remaining two fillets and one tablespoon oil. Add one fourth teaspoon pepper and ½ teaspoon salt evenly to cooked fillets.

- Step 4: Cleanse the skillet in step four. Heat the skillet over the medium-high heat with the remaining 1 1/2 teaspoons of oil. Add the chard and simmer it for three to four minutes, stirring periodically, until just barely soft.
- Step 5: Include the garlic and heat, frequently stirring, until it fragrant, about a minute. Cook for approximately a minute, occasionally stirring, after adding the lemon juice and wine.
- Step 6: Add the remaining 1/4 tsp. of salt and 1/4 tsp. of pepper before stirring in the butter. On top of the fish fillets, evenly distribute the chard mixture among the four dishes. Lemon wedges are optional.

Nutrition Facts

Calories: 368, carbohydrates: 6g, protein: 27g, fat: 25g

Chapter 4: Recipes of dinner

1: Italian Wedding Soup

Cook time: 18 min

Total time: 20 min

Servings: 6

Ingredients

- ⅔ cup of carrot (chopped)
- ½ teaspoon of salt (kosher)
- 4 cups of baby spinach
- 2 tablespoons of minced garlic
- 6 cups of chicken broth (unsalted)
- 1 ⅓ cup of yellow onion (chopped)
- ¼ cup of Parmesan cheese (grated)
- 1 ½ tablespoon of fresh oregano (chopped)
- 4 tablespoons of olive oil (extra-virgin)

- 6 ounces of orzo,(preferably whole-wheat)
- ⅔ cup of celery (chopped)
- 24 (12 ounces) chicken meatballs (cooked)

Directions

- Step 1: Heat 1 tablespoon oil in a large pot over medium to high heat. Add onion, carrot, celery and garlic; cook, occasionally stirring, until the onion is translucent, 4 to 5 minutes.
- Step 2: Add broth, cover and bring to a boil. Add orzo, oregano and salt; cover and cook, occasionally stirring, until the orzo is just tender, about 9 minutes.
- Step 3: Stir in meatballs and spinach; cook until the meatballs are heated through and the spinach is wilted 2 to 4 minutes.
- Step 4: Serve sprinkled with cheese and drizzled with the remaining 3 tablespoons oil.

Nutrition Facts

Calories: 415, carbohydrates: 36.1g, protein: 26g, fat: 19g

2: Roasted Vegetable & Black Bean Tacos

Cook time: 09 min

Total time: 15 min

Servings: 2

Ingredients

- ¼ teaspoon of salt (kosher)
- 1 teaspoon of cumin (ground)
- ½ avocado, cut into 8 slices
- 1 teaspoon of chilli powder
- 1 cup of root vegetables (roasted)
- 1 lime, cut into wedges
- ½ teaspoon of coriander (ground)
- 2 teaspoons of olive oil (extra-virgin)
- ¼ teaspoon of pepper (ground)
- ½ cup of cooked or canned of black beans, rinsed

- 4 corn tortillas (lightly toasted or warmed)
- Chopped cilantro & salsa for garnish

Directions

- Step 1: In a saucepan, mix the vegetables (roasted root), cumin, beans, oil, coriander, salt, chilli powder, and pepper. Cook with the lid on for 6 to 8 minutes, or until well heated.
- Step 2: Among the tortillas, distribute the ingredients. Avocado on top Lime wedges are recommended. If desired, garnish with salsa and/or cilantro.

Nutrition Facts

Calories: 343, carbohydrates: 44.4g, protein: 7.9g, fat: 16.8g

3: Spinach & Artichoke Dip Pasta

Cook time: 20 min

Total time : 20 min

Servings: 4

Ingredients

- 2 teaspoons of garlic powder
- 4 ounces of cream cheese (chopped into chunks)
- ¼ teaspoon of pepper (ground)
- ¾ cup milk (reduced-fat)
- 8 ounces of rotini (whole-wheat)
- 1 package of baby spinach (roughly chopped)
- ½ cup of cheese (Parmesan)
- 1 can of artichoke hearts (cut, squeezed dry and rinsed)

Directions

- Step 1: Start by heating up some water in a big pot. Cook pasta as directed on the packet. Drain.
- Step 2: Place the saucepan over medium flame and add 1 tablespoon water along with the spinach. About two minutes of cooking time should be spent with only occasional stirring. Put into a small bowl.
- Step 3: Stir the milk and cream cheese into pan till cream cheese is melted.

- Step 4: Include Parmesan, pepper, and garlic powder; cook while stirring until bubbling and thickened.
- Step 5: Drain the spinach of as like liquid as you can. Pasta, artichokes, and drained spinach are all stirred into sauce. Warm during cooking.

Nutrition Facts

Calories: 371, carbohydrates: 56g, protein: 16.6g, fat: 9g

4: Spinach Stew and Hearty Chickpea

Cook time: 20 min

Total time: 30 min

Servings: 4

Ingredients

- ½ teaspoon of dried oregano
- 3 tablespoons of tomato paste
- 1 tablespoon of olive oil
- ½ teaspoon of red pepper (crushed)
- ¼ teaspoon of ground pepper
- 12 ounces of ground turkey (93%-lean)
- 1 onion (chopped)
- ⅛ teaspoon salt
- 2 cans of divided rinsed chickpeas (low-sodium)
- 2 carrots (diced)
- ½ teaspoon of fennel seeds, crushed
- Three cups of IQF spinach
- 4 cloves of minced garlic (or half tsp. powder of garlic)
- 1 (32 ounces) carton
- 4 cups of chicken broth (low-sodium)
- ¼ cup of cheese (grated Parmesan)

Directions

- Step 1: Use the fork or potato masher to mash one can of chickpeas. Set apart.
- Step 2: Over the medium heat, warm oil in the pot. Add the (crushed) red pepper oregano, turkey, and fennel seeds simmer for two to three minutes, stirring occasionally, till the turkey isn't any longer pink. Add the carrots, garlic, and onion (or powder of garlic); simmer for three to four minutes, stirring frequently, till aromatic and softened. Add the tomato paste and stir for thirty sec.
- Step 3: Put the whole chickpeas after mashing, broth, salt, and pepper to pot. Put the lid on and simmer. Lower the flame to cook and medium, covered, quick simmer for about 10 minutes, or until the veggies are soft and the flavours are well-balanced.
- Step 4: Increase the flame to the medium-high before adding spinach. Cook the spinach for one to two minutes while stirring often. Into bowls, ladle soup. If preferred, top each plate with one Tablespoon. of Parmesan cheese.

Nutrition Facts

Calories: 401, carbohydrates: 41g, protein: 33.4g, fat: 13.4g

5: 20-Minute Balsamic Mushroom & Spinach Pasta

Cook time: 18 min

Total time: 20 min

Servings: 6

Ingredients

- 1 ½ tablespoon of garlic (thinly sliced)
- 3 tablespoons of balsamic vinegar
- ¾ teaspoon of salt
- 4 tablespoons of olive oil (extra-virgin)
- ½ teaspoon of ground pepper
- 3 ounces of baby spinach (about 3 cups)
- 8 ounces (whole-wheat) fettuccine or linguine
- ¼ cup fresh basil (chopped)
- 1 pound of cremini mushrooms, sliced (about 6 cups)
- 2 teaspoons of Worcestershire sauce, preferably vegetarian
- 6 tablespoons of unsalted pistachios (chopped roasted)

Directions

- Step 1: A big pot of water should first be brought to a boil. To prepare pasta, follow the instructions on the package. Save 1/4 cup of the cooking water before draining.
- Step 2: Heat 2 tablespoons of oil in a sizable nonstick skillet over medium to high heat in the meantime. When the mushrooms are added, simmer them for about 10 minutes while stirring occasionally. Add the garlic and continue to stir continuously for 30 seconds or so, until the garlic is aromatic. Add the spinach and boil it for a minute while stirring regularly.
- Step 3: Lower the heat to medium-low and add the Worcestershire, salt, pepper, and the remaining two tablespoons of oil. Pasta is added, then coated with a toss. Incorporate the 1/4 cup cooking water that was set aside. Leave the heat alone. Sprinkle pistachios on top after adding basil.

Nutrition Facts

Calories: 276, carbohydrates: 35g, protein: 10g, fat: 14g

6: Kale & Avocado Salad with Blueberries & Edamame

Cook time: 0 min

Total time: 20 min

Servings: 4

Ingredients

- ¼ cup of olive oil
- 1 cup of blueberries
- 1 ½ teaspoon of honey
- 1 teaspoon of Dijon mustard
- 1 avocado, diced
- 3 tablespoons juice of lemon
- 1 teaspoon of salt
- 1 cup of shelled edamame (cooked)
- 1 tablespoon of minced chives
- ¼ cup of sliced almonds, toasted
- 1 cup of cherry tomatoes(halved yellow)
- ½ cup of crumbled goat cheese (2 ounces)
- 6 cups of stemmed and curly kale (coarsely chopped)

Directions

- Step 1: Place the kale in a big bowl and knead the leaves with your hands to make them softer. Include avocado, tomatoes, blueberries, edamame, goat cheese, and almonds.
- Step 2: In a small bowl or jar with a secure lid, mix the lemon juice, oil, mustard, honey, and salt. Shake or whisk thoroughly.
- Step 3: Add the vinaigrette to the salad and toss to mix.

Nutrition Facts

Calories: 368, carbohydrates: 21g, protein: 10g, fat: 29g

7: One-Pot Lentil & Vegetable Soup with Parmesan

Cook time: 15 min

Total time: 40 min

Servings: 6

Ingredients

- ½ teaspoon of ground pepper
- ½ cup of cheese (grated Parmesan)
- Parmesan rind (optional)
- ½ teaspoon of salt
- ½ teaspoon of red pepper (crushed)
- 1 ½ cups of green or brown lentils
- 1 ½ tablespoon of vinegar (red wine)
- 4 cloves of garlic, chopped
- 2 tablespoons of olive oil (extra-virgin)
- 2 teaspoons of fresh thyme (finely chopped)
- Chopped parsley for garnish (fresh flat-leaf)
- 4 cups (low-sodium) vegetable or chicken broth
- 3 cups packed of lacinato kale (roughly chopped)
- 1 (15-ounce) can unsalted diced tomatoes, undrained
- 3 cups fresh or frozen chopped onion, carrot and celery mix

Directions

- Step 1: In a Dutch oven or big pot, heat the oil over medium heat. Add the mixture of onion, carrots, and celery; simmer for 6 to 10 minutes, stirring periodically, until softened. Add the garlic and simmer for 30 seconds, stirring frequently.
- Step 2: Add the broth, tomatoes, lentils, pepper, thyme, salt, red pepper (crushed), and, if using, the Parmesan rind. Stir to combine. Over medium to high heat, bring to a boil. Reduce the heat to medium-low; cover the pan and cook, stirring periodically, for 25 minutes, or until the lentils are almost cooked, adding water as necessary to thin to the desired consistency.
- Step 3: Add the kale. Cook the kale for 5 to 10 minutes under cover to make it soft. If using, remove and throw away the Parmesan rind. Vinegar should be added after

stirring. Six bowls should receive the soup; top with Parmesan. Adding parsley as a garnish is optional.

Nutrition Facts

Calories: 306, carbohydrates: 45g, protein: 17g, fat: 7g

8: Pinach & Artichoke Casserole with Chicken and Cauliflower Rice

Cook time: 20 min

Total time: 45 min

Servings: 4

Ingredients

- ½ cup of chicken broth (unsalted)
- 3 cups of fresh spinach (coarsely chopped)
- 1 ½ cups of Greek yoghurt (plain low-fat)
- ¼ teaspoon of ground pepper
- ¼ teaspoon of salt
- 2 cloves garlic, minced
- 4 cups of cauliflower rice (fresh or frozen)
- 1 tablespoon of olive oil (extra-virgin)
- 1 cup shredded mozzarella (part-skim)
- 1 (14 ounces) can of artichoke hearts, rinsed and chopped
- 1 pound of boneless, skinless chicken breasts, cut into bite-size pieces

Directions

- Step 1: To begin, preheat the oven to 375°F. Spray some cooking spray in a 9 by 13-inch baking dish.
- Step 2: In a big pot, heat the oil over medium heat. Add the chicken, season with salt and pepper, and stir-fry for about 8 minutes, or until the chicken is opaque on all sides. Add the garlic and stir for one minute. Get rid of the heat.
- Step 3: Pat artichokes dry in step three. Add 12 cups of dill Havarti, cauliflower rice, spinach, cream cheese and to the saucepan. Cream cheese should melt after being combined.

- Step 4: Move the mixture to the baking dish that has been prepared and top with the remaining 1/2 cup of dill Havarti. Bake for about 20 minutes or until the cheese is melted. Take it out of the oven, then stand there for five minutes. Dill should be added just before serving.

Nutrition Facts

Calories: 428, carbohydrates: 22g, protein: 39g, fat: 14g

9: Quinoa Chili with Sweet Potatoes

Cook time: 15 min

Total time: 30 min

Servings: 5

Ingredients

- 1 tablespoon of chilli powder
- 2 cups of water, divided
- 2 poblano peppers, diced
- 1 tablespoon of olive oil (extra-virgin)
- 4 cloves of garlic, chopped
- 1 (4 ounces) can of green chiles (diced)
- ½ teaspoon of salt
- 2 teaspoons of cumin (ground)
- 4 cups of vegetable broth (unsalted)
- 1 yellow onion, (medium diced)
- 1 cup of uncooked white or multicoloured quinoa
- 1 (15 ounces) can of pinto beans, (no-salt-added ,rinsed)
- 2 (12 ounces) sweet potatoes, peeled
- Sliced jalapeño peppers, yoghurt and cilantro for serving
- 1 (10 ounces) can no-salt-added diced tomatoes with green chiles

Directions

- Step 1: In the first step, warm the oil in a big saucepan over medium to high heat. Add the sweet potatoes and simmer, turning periodically, for 6 to 7 minutes until they are just starting to soften and brown. Add poblanos and onion; simmer, stirring occasionally, for about 3 minutes, or until onion is just beginning to soften.

- Step 2: Stir continuously for about 30 seconds while cooking the garlic, cumin, and chilli powder. Add 1 cup of water, the broth, the tomatoes, and the green chillies. Put a lid on it and heat it up to a rolling boil.
- Step 3: Add the quinoa, beans, and salt in step three. Reduce heat to medium, cover, and simmer the quinoa for 15 minutes or until it is cooked, stirring periodically. During the final 3 minutes of cooking, add the remaining 1 cup water.
- Step 4: Optional garnishes include yoghurt, cilantro, and jalapeno slices.

Nutrition Facts

Calories: 346, carbohydrates: 63g, protein: 12g, fat: 6g

10: Creamy Spinach Pasta

Cook time: 11 min

Total time: 15 min

Servings: 4

Ingredients

- 4 ounces of baby spinach
- ½ teaspoon of black pepper
- 2 tablespoons of shallots (thinly sliced)
- 3 ¼ ounces of mascarpone cheese
- 1 teaspoon of salt (kosher)
- 1 pinch of red pepper (Crushed)
- 1 clove of garlic, thinly sliced (about 1 tsp.)
- 1 teaspoon zest of lemon
- 12 ounces of chickpea pasta (uncooked tube-shaped)

Directions

- Step 1: First, prepare the pasta as directed on the package without adding salt. Drain while saving 1 cup of the cooking water.
- Step 2: Shift the pasta to the large bowl and add the spinach, garlic, mascarpone, shallot, salt, and pepper. Also, add half cup of the cooking liquid that was set aside.

For about 1 1/2 minutes, stir continuously till the cheese has melted and the mixture is mixed.

- Step 3: Add more cooking liquid if necessary to thin sauce. In four bowls, divide the spaghetti. Add some zest of lemon and (crushed) red pepper if you want. Serve instantly.

Nutrition Facts

Calories: 395, carbohydrates: 50g, protein: 23g, fat: 16g

11: One-Pot Lemon-Broccoli Pasta with Parmesan

Cook time: 20 min

Total time: 20 min

Servings: 4

Ingredients

- 1 ¾ cup of water
- 2 cloves of garlic, minced
- ½ teaspoon of salt
- 1 tablespoon zest of lemon
- ½ teaspoon of ground pepper
- 1 shallot, minced
- ⅓ cup of Parmesan cheese (grated)
- 8 ounces of farfalle pasta or rotini (whole-wheat)
- 4 teaspoons juice of lemon, or more to taste
- 2 tablespoons of olive oil (extra-virgin)
- 1 ½ cups of chicken broth or vegetable broth (low-sodium)
- 1 (10 ounces) of broccoli florets(frozen, thawed and chopped coarsely)

Directions

- Step 1: Warm the oil in the saucepan over the medium flame in the first step. For about two minutes, or until the shallot starts to soften, add it and stir. For about 30 seconds, while stirring, add the garlic and simmer until fragrant.

- Step 2: Add the lemon zest, water, broth, pepper pasta, and salt in step 2. Cover and heat until boiling. Cooking for 10 minutes at medium to high heat with frequent stirring requires removing the lid. Add the broccoli and often stir for two to three minutes, or till heated through.
- Step 3: Dish out and add lemon juice and Parmesan.

Nutrition Facts

Calories: 210, carbohydrates: 23g, protein: 9.3g, fat: 10.2g

12: Egg Drop Soup with Instant Noodles, Spinach & Scallions

Cook Time: 15 min

Total time: 20 min

Servings: 1

Ingredients

- 1 cup of baby spinach
- 2 cups of water
- 1 large egg
- 1 scallion, sliced
- ½ (3 ounces) package rice-noodle soup mix, such as Thai Kitchen Garlic & Vegetable

Directions

- Step 1: In a small saucepan, start by bringing water to a boil. Half of the seasoning packet should be mixed in (discard the remainder or reserve for another use). About 3 minutes after adding the noodles, they should be ready. Maintain a simmer by lowering the heat.
- Step 2: In a small bowl, whisk the egg. Stirring continuously, slowly add the egg to the soup that is simmering. Approximately 30 seconds after adding the spinach, fold it in.
- Step 3: Transfer to the bowl and top with scallions.

Nutrition Facts

Calories: 258, carbohydrates: 36.5g, protein: 10.9g, fat: 7.3g

13: Salt & Vinegar Sheet-Pan Chicken & Brussels Sprouts

Cook time: 20 min

Total time: 45 min

Servings: 4

Ingredients

- ½ teaspoon of dried dill
- ½ teaspoon of onion powder
- ½ teaspoon of garlic powder
- 1 teaspoon of kosher salt, divided
- ¼ teaspoon of sugar
- ½ teaspoon of ground pepper, divided
- 3 tablespoons of extra-virgin olive oil, divided
- 6 tablespoons of malt vinegar or sherry vinegar
- 1 ½ pounds bone-in, skin-on chicken breasts
- 2 medium red onions, cut into 1/2-inch wedges
- 1 ½ pound Brussels sprouts, trimmed and halved or quartered if large

Directions

- Step 1: Heat the oven to 450 degrees Fahrenheit.
- Step 2: Divide the chicken breasts into 4 equal pieces. Add one tablespoon of oil to the brush and 1⁄4 teaspoon of salt and pepper. Add the remaining Two tablespoons of oil, 1/4 teaspoon of salt, and 1⁄4 teaspoon of pepper to the big bowl of Brussels sprouts and onions. On a baking sheet with a rim, arrange the chicken, veggies, and other ingredients in a single layer.
- Step 3: Roast for 20 to 25 minutes, or until the veggies are soft and an instant-read thermometer inserted into the thickest part of a breast without touching bone reads 160 degrees Fahrenheit.
- Step 4: In the meantime, combine onion powder, vinegar, sugar, garlic powder, dill, sugar, and the final half teaspoon of salt in one small microwave-safe bowl. For about 30 seconds, on High, microwave the salt and sugar until they are dissolved.

- Step 5: Drizzle the vinegar mixture over the chicken and vegetables and roast for a further 5 minutes. As you toss the veggies in the skillet, remove the chicken from the pan and place it on a serving tray. Serve the chicken and veggies together.

Nutrition Facts

Calories: 387, carbohydrates: 19.9g, protein: 35.5g, fat: 18g

14: Avocado & Salmon Poke Bowl

Cook time: 20 min

Total time: 25 min

Servings: 4

Ingredients

For poke

- Half cup thinly sliced yellow onion
- Half cup chopped fresh cilantro
- One medium diced ripe avocado
- 2 teaspoons toasted (dark) sesame oil
- 3 tablespoons reduced-sodium tamari
- Half cup scallion greens (thinly sliced)
- Half teaspoon of Sriracha
- ¼ cup of tobiko or any other caviar (flying roe fish)
- 1 pound previously frozen wild salmon, skinned and cut into 3/4-inch cubes

For the Rice Salad

- Two tablespoons extra-virgin olive oil
- two cups of cooked warmed brown rice (short-grain)
- 1 tablespoon Chinese-style or Dijon mustard
- Two tablespoons rice vinegar
- 2 cups of spicy greens packed, such as mizuna or watercress and arugula

Directions

- Step 1: First, gently mix the avocado, salmon, onion, cilantro, scallion leaves, tobiko (or the caviar), sesame oil, tamari, and the Sriracha together in medium bowl.
- Step 2: The second step is to mix the rice with the greens in the big dish. In small bowl, combine the oil, vinegar, and mustard. Mix thoroughly after adding to rice salad. Rice salad should be served with the poke.

Nutrition Facts

Calories: 442, carbohydrates: 34.5g, protein: 29g, fat: 21g

15: Spinach, Lima Bean & Crispy Pancetta Pasta

Cook time: 20 min

Total time: 23 min

Servings: 4

Ingredients

- 1 cup of sliced shallots
- 4 cups of baby spinach
- 2 cloves of garlic, minced
- 3 tablespoons of lemon juice
- ½ teaspoon of dried rosemary
- 1 tablespoon olive oil (extra-virgin)
- ¾ cup of cheese (grated pecorino)
- 4 ounces diced pancetta
- 1 (9 ounces) package fresh spinach pasta
- 1 (16 ounces) package frozen baby lima beans, thawed

Directions

- Step 1: Heat up a medium saucepan of water to a rolling boil. Add the pasta and prepare it as directed on the package. Drain the pasta after saving 1 cup of the water.
- Step 2: In the meantime, warm the oil in a big skillet over medium to high heat. Pancetta should be added and cooked for 6 to 8 minutes, stirring periodically, until

crispy. To transfer to a plate, use a slotted spoon. To the pan, add shallots and lima beans. Shallots should be cooked for about 3 minutes, stirring regularly, until they are soft. Garlic and rosemary should be added after a minute or so of stirring until aromatic. After adding, boil the spinach for 2 minutes or until it wilts.

- Step 3: Add the pasta and the water that was set aside to the pan. About 1 minute of cooking and stirring is required to thicken the sauce. Lemon juice, pancetta, and half the pecorino are all added while stirring. Top the pasta with the rest of the pecorino.

Nutrition Facts

Calories: 477, carbohydrates: 61.6g, protein: 20.9g, fat: 16.2g

16: Roasted Root Veggies & Greens over Spiced Lentils

Cook time: 20 min

Total time: 45 min

Servings: 2

Ingredients

Lentils

- 1 teaspoon of garlic powder
- ¼ teaspoon of kosher salt
- ½ teaspoon of ground cumin
- 2 tablespoons juice of lemon
- 1 ½ cups of water
- ⅛ teaspoon of sumac (optional)
- ½ teaspoon of ground coriander
- 1 teaspoon of olive oil (extra-virgin)
- ¼ teaspoon of ground allspice
- ½ cup black beluga lentils or French green lentils

Vegetables

- One teaspoon of ground coriander
- One clove smashed garlic
- ⅛ teaspoon of ground pepper

- Pinch of kosher salt
- One and half cups of vegetables (roasted root)
- 1 tablespoon olive oil (extra-virgin)
- Fresh parsley for garnish
- 2 cups of chopped beet greens or kale
- 2 tablespoons of tahini or plain yoghurt (low-fat)

Directions

- Step 1: How to make lentils in step 1: In medium pot, combine garlic powder, water, lentils, ½ tsp. Each of coriander, cumin, and allspice, one fourth tsp. salt, and the sumac. Boiling is achieved. Cook for 25 to 30 minutes with the lid on, reducing heat to a simmer.
- Step 2: Remove the cover and continue cooking for another five min or so, or until liquid gradually decreases. Drain. Add 1 tsp. Oil and the lemon juice, stirring.
- Step 3: Steps to prepare the vegetables while waiting: Over medium heat, warm oil in one big skillet. Approximately one to two minutes later, add the garlic and heat it until fragrant. Add the root vegetables (roasted) and simmer, frequently stirring, for two to four minutes, or till it heated through. Kale (or the beet greens) should be added now and cooked for two to three minutes until barely wilted. Pepper, coriander, and the salt are stirred in.
- Step 4: Arrange the vegetables on top of the lentils and drizzle with the tahini (or the yoghurt). Adding parsley as a garnish is optional.

Nutrition Facts

Calories: 453, carbohydrates: 49.7g, protein: 18.1g, fat: 22.4g

17: Slow-Cooker Chicken & White Bean Stew

Cook time: 45 min

Total time: 7 hrs. 35 min

Servings: 6

Ingredients

- 4 cups of chopped kale
- ½ teaspoon of kosher salt
- 1 cup of sliced carrots
- 1 cup of yellow onion (chopped)
- ½ teaspoon of ground pepper
- 1 tablespoon juice of lemon
- 2 tablespoons olive oil (extra-virgin)
- 2 bone-in chicken breasts (1 pound each)
- 6 cups of chicken broth (unsalted)
- 1 teaspoon of fresh rosemary (finely chopped)
- ¼ cup of parsley leaves (flat-leaf)
- 1 pound dried cannellini beans, soaked overnight and drained
- 1 (4 ounces) Parmesan cheese rind plus 2/3 cup grated Parmesan, divided

Directions

- Step 1: A 6-quart slow cooker should be filled with the following ingredients: beans, onion, rosemary, broth, carrots, and Parmesan rind. Place chicken on top. Vegetables and beans should be cooked on Low for seven to eight hours with a cover on.
- Step 2: Transfer the chicken to a clean chopping board and leave it there for about 10 minutes or until it is safe to handle. Chicken should be shredded, bones removed.
- Step 3: The third step entails adding kale and adding the chicken back to the slow cooker. The kale should be soft after 20 to 30 minutes of cooking on High with the cover on.

- Step 4: Add the lemon juice, salt, and pepper; toss the Parmesan rind. Oil, Parmesan, and parsley should be added to the stew before serving.

Nutrition Facts

Calories: 493, carbohydrates: 55.8g, protein: 44.2g, fat: 10.9g

18: Sheet-Pan Chicken Fajita Bowls

Cook time: 20 min

Total time: 40 min

Servings: 4

Ingredients

- 2 teaspoons of chilli powder
- ¼ teaspoon of ground pepper
- 1 medium of yellow onion, sliced
- 2 tablespoons of olive oil, divided
- ¾ teaspoon of salt, divided
- 1 ¼ pound of chicken tenders
- 1 medium of red bell pepper, sliced
- 4 cups stemmed kale (chopped)
- ½ teaspoon of garlic powder
- ¼ cup of Greek yoghurt (low-fat plain)
- 1 medium green bell pepper, sliced
- 1 tablespoon of lime juice
- 2 teaspoons of ground cumin
- 2 teaspoons of water
- ½ teaspoon of smoked paprika
- 1 (15 ounce) can no-salt-added black beans, rinsed

Directions

- Step 1: Insert a sizable rimmed baking sheet into the oven, and heat it to 425 degrees Fahrenheit.
- Step 2: Mix the cumin, chilli powder, paprika, half teaspoon salt, garlic powder, and ground pepper in a big basin. Set aside a medium bowl with 1 teaspoon of the

spice mixture in it. In the big bowl, combine the remaining spice combination with 1 Tbsp. Oil. Toss the chicken, red and green bell peppers, onion, and dressing together.

- Step 3: Step three is to take the pan out of the oven and spray it with cooking spray. On the pan, evenly distribute the chicken mixture. 15 minutes of roasting.
- Step 4: In the meantime, combine the kale and black beans with the final 1/4 teaspoon of salt and 1 tablespoon of olive oil in a big bowl and toss to blend.
- Step 5: Take the pan out of the oven. The veggies and chicken are stirred. Beans and greens should be distributed evenly on top. For a further 5 to 7 minutes, roast the vegetables until they are soft and the chicken is thoroughly cooked.
- Step 6: Stir together the yoghurt, lime juice, and water before adding them to the spice combination that was set aside.
- Step 7: Distribute the chicken and vegetable combination among four bowls. After serving, drizzle with the yoghurt dressing.

Nutrition Facts

Calories: 343, carbohydrates: 25g, protein: 42.7g, fat: 9.9g

19: Slow-Cooker Mediterranean Diet Stew

Cook Time: 45 min

Total time: 6 hr. 45 min

Servings: 6

Ingredients

- ¾ cup of chopped carrot
- ¾ teaspoon of salt
- 1 teaspoon of dried oregano
- 1 tablespoon of lemon juice
- 1 cup of onion (coarsely chopped)
- 3 tablespoons of olive oil (extra-virgin)
- ¼ teaspoon of ground pepper
- Fresh basil leaves, torn if large
- 4 cloves garlic, minced
- 3 cups vegetable broth (low-sodium)
- 1 (15 ounce) can no-salt-added chickpeas, rinsed, divided
- ½ teaspoon red pepper (crushed)
- 6 lemon wedges (Optional)
- 1 bunch lacinato kale, stemmed and chopped (about 8 cups)
- 2 (14 ounce) cans no-salt-added fire-roasted diced tomatoes

Directions

- Step 1: In Step 1, combine the following ingredients in a slow cooker (4-quart): tomatoes, onion, broth, carrot, oregano, garlic, salt, red pepper (crushed), and pepper. Cook for 6 hours on Low with a cover on.
- Step 2: Measure 1/4 of the slow cooker's cooking liquid into a small basin in step 2. With a fork, mash 2 tablespoons of chickpeas until they are smooth.
- Step 3: To the mixture in the slow cooker, add the remaining whole chickpeas, mashed chickpeas, greens, and lemon juice. Blend by stirring. Kale takes around 30 minutes to get tender when covered and cooked on Low.
- Step 4: Evenly distribute the stew among 6 bowls and top with oil. Basil is a good garnish. If preferred, serve with lemon wedges.

Nutrition Facts

Calories: 191, carbohydrates: 22.9g, protein: 5.7g, fat: 7.8g

Chapter 5: Recipes of Drinks

1: Chocolate Nutter Butter Smoothie

Cook time: 0 min

Total time: 2 min

Servings: 1

Ingredients

- 1 scoop of Chocolate Protein Powder
- 2 tbsp of Pecans
- 1 medium banana (frozen)
- 1 cup of Spinach, Raw
- 3 Ice Cube
- 1 cup of Kefir (Nonfat Plain)
- 1 tbsp of Cacao Powder (Raw Organic)

Directions

- Step 1: Add banana, cacao powder, kefir, protein powder, pecans, ice cubes, spinach, and water to blender. Add some water depending on desired consistency.
- Step 2: Blend on high until mixture achieves a smooth consistency.

Nutrition Facts

Calories: 454, carbohydrates: 50g, protein: 37g, fat: 12g

2: Really Green Smoothie

Cook Time: 0 min

Total time: 5 min

Servings: 1

Ingredients

- 1 tablespoon of chia seeds

- 1 cup of ice cubes
- 1 cup of vanilla almond milk (unsweetened)
- ¼ ripe avocado
- 1 ripe banana
- 2 teaspoons of honey
- 1 cup of packed baby kale or coarsely chopped mature kale

Directions

- Step 1: In the blender, combine the kale, banana, almond milk, chia seeds, avocado, and honey.
- Step 2: Blend at a high speed until smooth and creamy. Blend in ice and till smooth.

Nutrition Facts

Calories: 343, carbohydrates: 54.7g, protein: 6g, fat: 14.2g

3: Mango & Kale Smoothie

Cook time: 0 min

Total time: 10 min

Servings: 1

Ingredients

- 1 small banana, sliced
- 1 cup frozen mango chunks
- 1 cup fresh orange juice
- 1 cup baby kale

Directions

- Step 1: First, fill up the blender with the mango, kale, banana, and the orange juice. Blend until it is well combined at the medium speed, using up the tamper in case if it is required.
- Step 2: Boost the speed to the medium-high, then blend until the mixture is very smooth.

Nutrition Facts

Calories: 329, carbohydrates: 82g, protein: 4g, fat: 1g

4: Cherry-Mocha Smoothie

Cook time: 0 min

Total time: 10 min

Servings: 2

Ingredients

- One cup milk of chocolate almond (unsweetened)
- 1 teaspoon of vanilla
- ½ banana (medium)
- Two tablespoons of almond butter
- One teaspoon of coffee powder (instant espresso)
- 2 tablespoons of cocoa powder (unsweetened)
- 2 cups of ice cubes
- 1 cup of dark sweet cherries (frozen unsweetened pitted)
- 5.3 to 6-ounce of carton vanilla (fat-free Greek yoghurt)
- 1 tablespoon of chocolate shavings, espresso beans (chocolate-covered)

Directions

- Step 1: Blend the almond milk, cocoa powder, cherries, almond butter, banana, Greek yoghurt, vanilla, and the coffee powder (espresso) together in a blender. Until smooth, blend and cover.
- Step 2: Incorporate the ice cubes, cover, and blend until smooth. Pour into the glasses and, if preferred, top with more banana slices, chocolate shavings, or espresso beans (chocolate-covered).

Nutrition Facts

Calories: 272, carbohydrates: 34g, protein: 13g, fat: 12g

5: Strawberry-Almond Smoothie

Cook time: 0 min

Total time: 10 min

Servings: 2

Ingredients

- 10 whole strawberries (frozen)
- 1/2 cup of silken tofu, (4 ounces)
- 1 cup of almond milk or low-fat milk
- 2 tablespoons of sugar

Directions

- Step 1: In the first step, mix the almond milk, strawberries, sugar, and tofu (or low-fat milk).
- Step 2: Blend for about a minute, until it is smooth and frothy. Serve the mixture in large glasses.

Nutrition Facts

Calories: 171, carbohydrates: 30.4g, protein: 4.6g, fat: 3.3g

6: Blueberry & Avocado Smoothie

Cook time: 0 min

Total time: 10 min

Servings: 1

Ingredients

- ½ avocado, pitted and sliced
- 1 cup of vanilla coconut milk (unsweetened)
- 5 dates (pitted and roughly chopped)
- 1 cup of frozen blueberries

Directions

- Step 1: Blend in a blender dates, avocado, blueberries, and coconut milk. Blend until well combined at medium-low speed, using tamper if it is required.
- Step 2: Boost the speed to the medium-high, then blend until the mixture is very smooth.

Nutrition Facts

Calories: 405, carbohydrates: 59g, protein: 4g, fat: 20g

7: Spinach Smoothie

Cook time: 0 min

Total time: 10 min

Servings: 1

Ingredients

- 1 ½ cup of baby spinach
- 1 cup of frozen strawberries
- 1 small of banana, sliced
- 6 of cups unsweetened vanilla coconut milk or other non-dairy milk

Directions

- Step 1: Blend spinach, coconut milk, strawberries, banana, and any other milk of your choice. As needed, use up the tamper while blending on medium-low speed to ensure thorough blending.
- Step 2: Increase the speed to medium-high and blend until extremely smooth.

Nutrition Facts

Calories: 183, carbohydrates: 39g, protein: 4g, fat: 4g

8: Kale & Pineapple Smoothie

Cook Time: 0 min

Total time: 10 min

Servings: 1

Ingredients

- 1 cup of pineapple chunks (frozen)
- 1 cup of baby kale
- ½ cup of orange juice (fresh)
- ¼ cup of plain or coconut Greek yoghurt
- ½ cup vanilla coconut milk (unsweetened)

Directions

- Step 1: Blend up the kale with the yoghurt, pineapple, coconut milk, and orange juice. Use the tamper if required and blend until well blended at medium-low speed.
- Step 2: Increase speed to medium-high and continue blending till very smooth.

Nutrition Facts

Calories: 231, carbohydrates: 41g, protein: 9g, fat: 3g

9: Spinach-Avocado Smoothie

Cook time: 0 min

Total time: 5 min

Servings: 1

Ingredients

- 1 frozen banana
- 2 tablespoons of water
- 1 cup of fresh spinach
- ¼ avocado
- 1 teaspoon of honey
- 1 cup plain yoghurt (nonfat)

Directions

- Step 1: Blend water, yoghurt, banana, spinach, avocado, and the honey. Blend in a blender until completely smooth.

Nutrition Facts

Calories: 357, carbohydrates: 57.8g, protein: 17.7g, fat: 8.2g

10: Kale & Spinach Smoothie

Cook time: 0 min

Total time: 10 min

Servings: 1

Ingredients

- 1 kiwi, peeled and sliced
- 1 cup of baby spinach
- 2 tablespoons of almond butter(creamy)
- 1 cup of baby kale
- 5 dates, pitted and roughly chopped
- 1 cup of vanilla almond milk (unsweetened)

Directions

- Step 1: Blend together spinach, kale, dates, almond milk, kiwi, and all of the mentioned ingredients. As needed, use the tamper while blending on the medium or low speed to ensure thorough blending.
- Step 2: Increase the speed to the medium-high and then blend until extremely smooth.

Nutrition Facts

Calories: 419, carbohydrates: 51g, protein: 12g, fat: 21g

11: Turmeric Latte

Cook time: 5 min

Total time: 5 min

Servings: 2

Ingredients

- 1 tsp. of Spices, cardamom
- 1 tsp. of Rose Water
- 3/5 g Pepper, Ground Black
- 1 tsp. of Turmeric
- 1 tsp. of Honey (Organic raw)
- 2 1/2 cups of Almond Breeze, Almond Coconut Blend

Directions

- Step 1: Combine all the ingredients in a sauce pan and simmer the mixture over low heat.
- Step 2: Whisk occasionally.

- Step 3: Distribute equally between the two mugs, garnish according to your liking, and enjoy.
- Step 4: Optional garnishes, including cacao nibs, ground cardamom, crushed rose petals (dried), sesame seeds, chopped almonds, and turmeric

Nutrition Facts

Calories: 64, carbohydrates: 1g, protein: 2g, fat: 4g

12: Berry Green Smoothie

Cook time: 0 min

Total time: 10 min

Servings: 1

Ingredients

- 2 tablespoons of water
- 1 cup mixed berries (frozen)
- 1 ripe banana, sliced
- 1/2 cup of baby spinach leaves
- 2 tablespoons of orange juice (fresh)
- 1 (5.3-oz.) container plain 2% reduced-fat Greek yoghurt

Directions

- Step 1: Place all the ingredients in blender and process it until smooth.

Nutrition Facts

Calories: 29, carbohydrates: 54g, protein: 18g, fat: 3.8g

13: Orange-Mango Gritty with Turmeric and Walnuts

Cook time: 0 min

Total time: 10 min

Servings: 2

Ingredients

- 3/4 cup plain 2% reduced-fat Greek yoghurt
- 1 cup ice cubes

- 1 tablespoon ground flaxseed
- 1/2 cup orange slices (fresh)
- 1/4 cup orange juice (fresh)
- 2 teaspoons of turmeric (grated fresh)
- 1/4 cup of toasted walnuts (chopped)
- Dash of kosher salt
- 3/4 cup ripe mango (frozen chopped peeled)
- Freshly grated nutmeg (optional)

Directions

- Step 1: Put the first nine ingredients in the blender and blend for one minute or until nearly smooth. Between two glasses, divide the mixture equally. If desired, grate some nutmeg on top.

Nutrition Facts

Calories: 245, carbohydrates: 25g, protein: 11g, fat: 13.1g

14: Banana-Pineapple-Kale Smoothie

Cook Time: 0 min

Total time: 5 min

Servings: 2

Ingredients

- 1/2 cup of pineapple cubes (fresh)
- 1 small frozen banana
- 1 cup of baby kale (1 ounce)
- 1/3 cup of coconut milk (light)

Directions

- Step 1: Blend the all ingredients for about thirty seconds, or until they are completely smooth. Serve right away.

Nutrition Facts

Calories: 166, carbohydrates: 37g, protein: 4g, fat: 2g

15: Green Tea and Ginger Tonic

Cook time: 5 min

Total time: 5 min

Servings: 2

Ingredients

- 4 leaves of mint
- 2 cups of water
- 2 green tea bags
- 2 tablespoons of minced ginger (with skins on)
- 2 teaspoons honey, divided
- 1/8 teaspoon of cayenne pepper

Directions

- Step 1: Put mint leaves, honey, and tea bags (green tea) in 2 glasses.
- Step 2: Bring water, cayenne, and ginger to the rolling boil in one small saucepot. Divide tea into 2 glasses after straining through a mesh sieve. Remove the tea bag and the mint leaves after three minutes of steeping to drink.

Nutrition Facts

Calories: 22, carbohydrates: 5g, protein: 0g, fat: 0g

Chapter 6: Recipes of Snacks

1: Chocolate-Peanut Butter Energy Bars

Cook time: 5 min

Total time: 1 hr. 25 min

Servings: 16

Ingredients

- ¾ cup of Medjool dates (chopped)
- ¼ teaspoon of salt
- ½ cup of rolled oats
- ½ cup of peanuts dry-roasted (chopped unsalted)
- 1 cup of peanut butter (smooth natural)
- ¾ cup chocolate chips (bittersweet)

Directions

- Step 1: For ten min, cover dates with hot water in medium bowl. Drain and keep soaking water aside.
- Step 2: In the meantime, line a baking pan that is 8 inches squares with the parchment paper, leaving the extra hanging over the two sides. Cooking spray should be lightly applied to the parchment.
- Step 3: Place the oats, salt, soaked dates and peanut butter in a food processor; pulse until the mixture is very finely minced and beginning to clump. Add a few tablespoons at a time of the saved soaking water if the mixture feels dry. Add peanuts after transferring to a medium bowl. The ingredients should be pressed firmly and evenly into prepared pan.
- Step 4: Microwave the chocolate chips in one microwave-safe container for two to three minutes on the Medium (50%) till melted. Over the mixture of oat, cover it completely with chocolate. About an hour will pass while the food is being chilled in the refrigerator. By raising the dangling parchment, remove from pan. Square up into sixteen pieces.

Nutrition Facts

Calories: 203, carbohydrates: 17.4g, protein: 5.4g, fat: 12.7g

2: Avocado Hummus

Cook time: 0 min

Total time: 10 min

Servings: 10

Ingredients

- 1 ripe avocado, halved and pitted
- 1 clove garlic
- 1 teaspoon ground cumin
- ¼ cup lemon juice
- ½ teaspoon salt
- 1 cup fresh cilantro leaves
- ¼ cup extra-virgin olive oil
- ¼ cup tahini
- 1 (15 ounce) can no-salt-added chickpeas

Directions

- Step 1: Chickpeas should be drained with two tablespoons of liquid saved. Add the chickpeas and the liquid you set aside to the food processor. Avocado, cilantro, oil, tahini, lemon juice, cumin, garlic, and the salt should all be added till very smooth, pure. Serve with crudités, vegetable chips or pita chips.

Nutrition Facts

Calories: 156, carbohydrates: 9.5g, protein: 3.3g, fat: 12.4g

3: Chocolate and Strawberry Greek Yogurt Bark

Cook time: 10 min

Total time: 3 hrs. 10 min

Servings: 32

Ingredients

- ¼ cup of maple syrup or honey
- 1 ½ cup sliced strawberries
- 1 teaspoon vanilla extract
- ¼ cup chocolate chips (mini)

- 3 cups whole-milk plain Greek yoghurt

Directions

- Step 1: Put parchment paper along the edge of a baking pan.
- Step 2: In the medium bowl, combine yoghurt, vanilla, and maple syrup (or the honey). Shape ten- by fifteen-inch rectangle and spread out on the baking sheet that has been prepped. Add chocolate chips on top after scattering the strawberries.
- Step 3: For at least three hours, freeze until very solid. 32 pieces should be cut or broken off to serve.

Nutrition Facts:

Calories: 34, carbohydrates: 5g, protein: 2g, fat: 1.3g

4: Peanut Butter Energy Balls

Cook time: 0 min

Total time: 20 min

Servings: 17

Ingredients

- 2 cups of rolled oats
- ¼ cup of mini chocolate chips
- ½ cup of honey
- ¼ cup shredded coconut (unsweetened)
- 1 cup of natural peanut butter or other nut butter

Directions

- Step 1: In medium bowl, whisk together the oats, honey, peanut butter (or any nut butter), coconut, and chocolate chips. Make balls out of the mixture using a one-tablespoon measure. For a maximum of three months in the freezer or five days in the refrigerator, store in airtight container.

Nutrition Facts

Calories: 174, carbohydrates: 18.2g, protein: 4.4g, fat: 9.2g

5: Lemon-Blueberry Bars

Cook time: 30 min

Total time: 2 hrs. 40 min

Servings: 9

Ingredients

- ½ cup of lemon juice
- 1 tablespoon of granulated sugar
- 1 large egg
- 1 ¼ cup of graham cracker crumbs
- 1 cup of fresh blueberries
- Zest of 1 lemon, divided
- 4 tablespoons salted butter, melted
- 1 (14 ounces) can sweetened condensed milk

Directions

- Step 1: Set oven to 350 degrees Fahrenheit. Apply cooking spray to a baking dish that is 8 inches square.
- Step 2: Combine the sugar, butter, lemon zest, and graham cracker crumbs in a medium basin. In the prepared pan, press the ingredients firmly and uniformly. About 10 minutes of baking time will have the edges just barely browned. Allow to cool for at least 10 minutes in the pan on wire rack.
- Step 3: Lemon juice, condensed milk, egg, and the remaining of the lemon zest should all be thoroughly whisked together in medium bowl in the meantime. Blueberries have been added after stirring. Over the baked crust, spread the filling evenly. 16 - 18 minutes of baking time until set. Wait an hour for the room to cool. For at least another hour, cover and chill.

Nutrition Facts

Calories: 273, carbohydrates: 40g, protein: 5g, fat: 11g

6: Garlic Hummus

Cook time: 0 min

Total time: 10 min

Servings: 8

Ingredients

- ¼ cup of olive oil (extra-virgin)
- ¼ cup of tahini
- 1 clove garlic
- ½ teaspoon of chili powder
- ¼ cup of lemon juice
- ½ teaspoon of salt
- 1 teaspoon of ground cumin
- 1 (15 ounce) can no-salt-added chickpeas

Directions

- Step 1: Chickpeas should be drained with 1 tbsp. of liquid saved. Add all chickpeas and the liquid you set aside to food processor.
- Step 2: Tahini, lemon juice, oil, garlic, chilli powder, cumin, and the salt are added in step 2. Puree for two to three minutes or until extremely smooth.

Nutrition Facts

Calories: 155, carbohydrates: 9.7g, protein: 3.7g, fat: 11.9g

7: Almost Chipotle's Guacamole

Cook time: 0 min

Total time: 15 min

Servings: 8

Ingredients

- ¼ cup of fresh cilantro (chopped)
- 1 clove garlic, grated
- 1 medium jalapeño pepper, finely chopped
- 2 tablespoons of lime juice
- 3 medium ripe avocados

- ½ teaspoon of salt
- ¼ cup of red or white onion (finely chopped)

Directions

- Step 1: With a fork, mash the avocados in medium basin. Stir in the jalapenos, onions, cilantro, lime juice, garlic, and salt after adding them.

Nutrition Facts

Calories: 125, carbohydrates: 7.5g, protein: 1.6g, fat: 11.1g

8: Peanut Butter Blueberry Energy Balls

Cook time: 0 min

Total time: 20 min

Servings: 17

Ingredients

- 2 cups rolled oats
- ¼ cup mini chocolate chips
- ½ cup honey
- ¼ cup dehydrated blueberries
- 1 cup natural peanut butter or other nut butter

Directions

- Step 1: In medium bowl, whisk together the honey, oats, peanut butter (you can use any nut butter of your choice), blueberries, and chocolate chips. Make balls out of the mixture using 1 tablespoon measure. For a maximum of three months in freezer or five days in refrigerator, store in the airtight container.

Nutrition Facts

Calories: 183, carbohydrates: 20g, protein: 5g, fat: 9g

9: Raspberry-Lemon Greek Frozen Yogurt Bark

Cook time: 0 min

Total time: 3 hrs. 15 min

Servings: 16

Ingredients

- 2 tablespoons of lemon juice
- ¼ cup of honey
- 1 teaspoon of vanilla extract
- 3 cups of Greek yoghurt (whole-milk plain)
- Zest of 1 lemon
- 6 ounces raspberries, halved lengthwise

Directions

- Step 1: Spread parchment paper down the edge of a sizable baking sheet.
- Step 2: The second step is to combine the lemon juice, yoghurt, honey, and vanilla in a medium bowl. Form a 10 by 15-inch rectangle and spread out on the baking sheet that has been prepped. Lemon zest should be added along with the raspberries.
- Step 3: Freeze for a minimum of three hours, or until very firm. 32 pieces should be cut or broken off to serve.

Nutrition Facts

Calories: 69, carbohydrates: 8g, protein: 5g, fat: 3g

10: Roasted Buffalo Chickpeas

Cook time: 35 min

Total time: 45 min

Servings: 4

Ingredients

- 1 tablespoon of white vinegar
- ¼ teaspoon of salt
- ½ teaspoon of cayenne pepper, or to taste
- 1 (15 ounce) can no-salt-added chickpeas, rinsed

Directions

- Step 1: First, place the oven rack in the highest third and preheat the oven to the 400 degrees Fahrenheit.
- Step 2: Mix salt, cayenne, and vinegar in a sizable bowl. After carefully patting the chickpeas dry, combine the mixture of the vinegar with them. On the baking sheet with a rim, spread.
- Step 3: Roast up the chickpeas in the oven for thirty to thirty-five minutes, turning them twice, until they are crisp and golden. For thirty min, let the chickpeas cool on the pan; as they cool, they will become crisp.

Nutrition Facts

Calories: 109, carbohydrates: 17.6g, protein: 5.8g, fat: 0.9g

Conclusion

The protective effects of inflammation also help the body withstand illness. It typically marks a critical point in the healing process.

However, in some individuals, an underlying medical problem stops the immune system from operating normally. Low-grade inflammation that is persistent or recurrent could result from this dysfunction.

Asthma, rheumatoid arthritis, and psoriasis are a few of the diseases that cause persistent inflammation. There is proof that changing one's diet can help manage symptoms.

Anti-inflammatory diets promote the consumption of vegetables, fruits, and meals high in fatty acids (omega-3), lean protein, whole grains, healthy fats, and spices. It restricts or discourages the eating of red meat, alcohol, and processed foods.

Anti-inflammatory diet is more of a way of eating than a particular diet. For instance, DASH diet and Mediterranean diet both lower inflammation.

Fresh fruits and vegetables make up the majority of an anti-inflammatory diet. Antioxidants are plentiful in plant-based meals. Some compounds, however, can actually cause the production of free radicals. Foods that are continuously fried in hot oil are examples.

Antioxidant chemicals included in food aid in the body's removal of free radicals. Free radicals are the results of several physiological functions that the body naturally performs, including metabolism. However, two examples of external stressors that may raise the body's levels of free radicals include stress and smoking.

Cells can suffer damage from free radicals. This damage makes inflammation more likely and could contribute to numerous ailments.

In addition to the antioxidants, the body naturally produces dietary antioxidants that aid in the removal of these harmful substances.

Foods that lower the formation of free radicals is preferred in anti-inflammatory diets over those that are high in antioxidants.

THIS BOOK INCLUDES FREE BONUSES

THESE BONUSES ARE 100% FREE. AND ALL YOU NEED TO GET IT IS A NAME AND AN EMAIL ADDRES! IT'S SUPER EASY!

DIET JOURNAL

SCAN ME

60 DAYS MEAL PLAN

Printed in Great Britain
by Amazon

22864989R00057